OTHERS' MILK

OTHERS' MILK

The Potential of
Exceptional Breastfeeding

KRISTIN J. WILSON

Dear Sally,
So happy to
know another comrade
who believes in community !
Love,

RUTGERS UNIVERSITY PRESS

New Brunswick, Camden, and Newark, New Jersey, and London

Library of Congress Cataloging-in-Publication Data

Names: Wilson, Kristin J., 1972–
Title: Others' milk : the potential of exceptional breastfeeding / Kristin J. Wilson.
Description: New Brunswick : Rutgers University Press, 2018. | Includes
bibliographical references and index.
Identifiers: LCCN 2017056013 | ISBN 9780813593845 (hardback) |
ISBN 9780813593838 (paperback)
Subjects: LCSH: Breastfeeding. | Breastfeeding—Social aspects. | BISAC:
HEALTH & FITNESS / Breastfeeding. | FAMILY & RELATIONSHIPS /
Parenting / Child Rearing. | SOCIAL SCIENCE / Women's Studies. | SOCIAL
SCIENCE / Gender Studies. | MEDICAL / Nursing / Maternity, Perinatal, Women's
Health. | SOCIAL SCIENCE / Lesbian Studies. | SOCIAL SCIENCE / Sociology /
Marriage & Family.
Classification: LCC RJ216 .W683 2018 | DDC 649/.33—dc23
LC record available at https://lccn.loc.gov/2017056013

A British Cataloging-in-Publication record for this book is available from the British
Library.

∞ The paper used in this publication meets the requirements of the American
National Standard for Information Sciences—Permanence of Paper for Printed
Library Materials, ANSI Z39.48-1992.

www.rutgersuniversitypress.org

Manufactured in the United States of America

CONTENTS

OTHERS' MILK

1 · NURSING IS PUBLIC

A hungry baby cries in the night. Still dreaming, Cory momentarily tries to block out the distressing sound by burrowing into the pillow but then starts awake. With only a little reluctance, the routine begins: trudging out of bed, wriggling out of a pajama top that no longer quite fits, and shuffling across the room over to the crib. Baby Ella begins to quiet as soon as she sees Cory, more so when she is embraced and held close against a warm chest. Doing as babies instinctively do, she begins to root for milk, finding the nipple and, full of trust, locking eyes with her . . . big brother.

Cory is a typical ten-year-old American boy in most ways. He goes to school and hangs out with friends. He also "nurses" his baby sister; they call it *on-sies*. I asked his mother, Lanie, if this term meant that the baby was "on," but she told me it might be a little one's mispronunciation of *nursies*, the term her older children once used. To her, a de facto excommunicated La Leche League leader—her definitions do not meet with their doctrines—it means nursing and, to her, nursing means the loving delivery of sustenance, preferably breast milk, to an infant. Cory does on-sies by holding a bottle of breast milk at his chest for his sister while Lanie cares for an even younger sibling who has severe health problems.

When the foster care system first placed Ella with their family, Lanie induced lactation and breastfed her for a few months. Inducing lactation is no easy task. It requires a great deal of pumping, frequent suckling, and sometimes the use of certain medications. Breastfeeding foster children is only permissible with a judge's order, which takes too long to get (several weeks to months, depending on the court schedule). Lanie believes that all children deserve the opportunity to breastfeed if possible, so she does it anyway and keeps it quiet. Breastfeeding a foster baby can be grounds for removing a child; this strictness is ostensibly due to fears of HIV transmission but probably also has to do with cultural assumptions about entwined mother-baby relationships and with institutions' habitual need to engage in surveillance.

When a judge deemed Ella's struggling birth mother ready to care for her infant, Lanie's family received a mere few hours' warning that baby and birth mother would be reunited. The court order threw the family into an emotional crisis, but Cory seemed unsettlingly unaffected—Lanie thought, "Note to self: work on empathy with this kid." But he turned from his Legos and calmly explained, "Mommy, if you needed a second chance to have me back, I would want you to have it because you are my best mommy ever." This comment remained a touchstone for Lanie through the months without Ella. She decided that she would root for the birth mother to obtain the support that she needed to get her life together and tried to appreciate the precious time they all shared with the baby.

Sadly, despite good intentions, Ella's birth mother failed to stay off drugs. A few months later, the baby experienced terrible trauma at the breast when her mother had a sudden, near-fatal, drug-related cardiac event. Someone called 9-1-1, and the paramedics saved Ella and her birth mother. Social workers reentered the picture. Ella was returned to Cory's family just as suddenly as she had left. By then, a new foster baby, Lydia, had joined the family. She was a tiny preemie who had arrived with a surprising amount of medical equipment and a long list of instructions from the hospital.

Ella had changed in her months away. She became unwilling to nurse and was distressed even when being held. She wailed and shrieked, only to act listless in turns. Through torturous days and nights of trial and error, trying every trick in every book, Lanie and her husband found some success with kangaroo care. *Kangaroo care* refers to skin-to-skin contact, which is often recommended these days by hospitals and medical providers as a way to care for premature babies and as a way to promote lactation. The baby is usually only clad in a diaper, the caregiver is bare-chested, and the baby is in a sling or wrap. This skin-to-skin contact promotes sharing warmth and the feeling of one another's heartbeats. It feels good and snuggly. Anyone can do it. And so Cory, who loves having Ella back and whose summer plans amount to playing video games and Legos, coos to his foster sister as he holds her close and gives her a bottle of donated breast milk that his dad drove an hour to get from a generous pumping mother who

Lanie met online. Lanie attends to her youngest child, Lydia, who gets her nourishment—special formula mixed with donated milk—through a GI (gastrointestinal) tube.

The circumstances of this family's story may be particular, but the sentiments that guide them are not. They love each other and support each other in getting their youngest members' needs met. Lanie boasts that when her other children heard that Ella was coming back, their first collective thought was "Let's hop in the car and get some breast milk!" She laughs that her husband advised everyone in the family to "slow down!"—"The first need [cue anticipation-filled pause] is a car seat," he told them, tongue in cheek. For this family, nourishing a foster child means acquiring donated milk. "That is who we are," Lanie declares. Getting milk means piling in the car and traveling miles on the interstate to meet up with a trusted stranger offering a cooler full of pumped milk. They usually arrange to meet up in a Walmart or drugstore parking lot off of an exit ramp. This drive (in both senses of the word) to get a baby breastfed, by whatever means they can, follows a consistent logic shared by a diverse swath of loving caregivers. They are "exceptional breastfeeders."[1]

OTHERS' MILK

I mean *Others' Milk*, the title of this book, as a triple entendre. The more common phrase, "mother's milk," implies that breastfeeding is individual, essential, and natural. The experience, though, is very much a social one—a fact made obvious by exceptional breastfeeding.

The mothers in this book provide breast milk and suckle babies, while the "others" encompass a much wider group who include Cory the son, friends who take turns nursing one another's babies so they can still go to their paid jobs, transmasculine "chestfeeding" parents, and the modern-day wet nurses who provide enhanced day care that includes breastfeeding. Adoptive and foster mothers, relational mothers by virtue of surrogacy, and nongestational mothers in lesbian partnerships or marriages may also breastfeed and/or provide breast milk. The phrase "mother's milk" makes it sound like the breastfeeder gestated and birthed the nursling, but this is clearly not always the case.

Others' Milk also refers to the phenomenon in which many milk donors begin to see their pumped milk as already belonging to others. Barbara Katz

Rothman points out that the very term *breastfeeding* puts the focus on the milk rather than on the ongoing relationship between mother and baby.[2] This existing framework makes it ever easier to conceive of milk as a product that belongs to someone other than the producer. First, it belongs to the baby, and then, thanks to the pump, it can belong to anyone. Someone who is lactating may pump for other mothers who they see as much like themselves, or they may imagine saving babies with their extra pumping sessions. Some hold both thoughts in mind, and still others just want to get rid of the extra bags crowding their freezers. One woman told me that she needed to make room for "hubby's ice cream." Yet throwing out freezer stashes does not occur without a hefty measure of consternation and sometimes even grief. The milk itself is imbued with labor and love;[3] some even see it as going through an almost holy transubstantiation from bodily fluid to life-giving ambrosia. Intent is the magical ingredient in this alchemical process that converts breast milk into what many call "liquid love" or, more frequently, "liquid gold." To be sure, some breastfeeders see donation of their surplus as a good citizen's household duty, like recycling. In either framework, caregivers providing their babies with donated milk are giving them "others' milk."

Finally, *Others' Milk* is about how we as a society regard others' choices about infant and toddler nourishment and nurturance. Social strictures shape what we believe to be private decisions for ourselves and for our families. Hospital protocols, how-to guides, and other experts strongly influence parents' "breastfeeding style," a concept that refers to the timing of breastfeeding initiation, the frequency of feeds, and so on.[4] The medical model of breastfeeding often centers on the baby and focuses on the production and quality of the breast milk—but not on the breastfeeders' holistic experience.[5] And yet others' milk seems to be everyone's business.

The public discusses all aspects of breastfeeding in thoroughly moralistic and medicalized ways. People share video clips on social media of women being berated by strangers for nursing in public. Though preposterous, commenters on the internet commonly compare breastfeeding in public to urinating in public as a retort to the explanation that "it is natural." Facebook frequently freezes the accounts of those who post pics of themselves nursing—reportedly even with no nipple in view—as a violation of their "community standards" of modesty. The May 10, 2012, cover of *Time*, depicting a toddler standing on a stool to nurse, reached instant infamy as an emblem of taking things too far. Those who do not breastfeed run the risk of public ire for lazily or selfishly giving their babies inferior sustenance and denying them a foundational bonding opportunity.[6] Our society monitors the breastfeeding choices of anyone and everyone including—but not limited to—mothers who wean so that they can return to paid jobs, who pump so that a hired caregiver can provide their milk in a bottle, and who lose footing in their careers by staying home to nurse on demand.

Those who do not breastfeed for whatever reason, especially middle-class white women, feel so judged and pressured that they may attempt to divert scorn by fooling observers. They may limit how often they leave home or, if they do go out in public, offer formula to their babies using bottles designed to attach to breast pumps. The pervasive "breast is best" motto comes with impossible caveats. Mothers should breastfeed—but not in public, not for too long, not in front of male family members, not while on medication, and the list goes on. Nearly everyone feels criticized and defensive, and this negativity feeds the media-stoked "mommy wars." The mommy wars are not really between mommies; they are manufactured, drummed-up public controversies that primarily impact mothers, who are always being blamed for societal ills.[7] A single outrageous incident can touch off op-ed battles and flame wars.[8] It's draining.

Those breastfeeders who find themselves *really* pushing the boundaries of breastfeeding—nursing their seven-year-old, being transgender and breastfeeding, nursing in church over protestations—not only have to navigate the standard-issue breastfeeding dilemmas but also find themselves disrupting taken-for-granted narratives. Their border-crossing experiences reveal moral paradoxes that undergird foundational social institutions like motherhood, kinship, and medicine.

On one hand, when all goes relatively well with breastfeeding, when it looks fairly normative, these institutions support breastfeeding and breastfeeding supports these institutions' objectives. It is expected of "good mothers" these days.[9] Good mothers breastfeed, and breastfeeding helps define motherhood by separating good mothers from the supposedly less-committed variety. Breastfeeding is seen not only as optimal nutrition but also as a way to solidify one's relationship with her baby.[10] The constant drip of scientific findings that breast milk contains ingredients tailor-made for each of a specific breastfeeder's own babies makes the relationship seem preordained. These ideas shore up a hierarchy of kinship that understands women as mothers first and foremost. It is a truism among breastfeeding researchers and advocates that the mother-baby bond represents the most basic and fundamental of human social relationships. One breast milk scientist is quoted as saying, "There is a connection between the mom and the infant that you just could not mimic in a bottle, in a powder."[11]

A common refrain in public health initiatives to increase breastfeeding initiation and duration rates is to better educate the medical team, perhaps by thoroughly "integrating" services between obstetrician (OB), pediatrician, and lactation consultant.[12] These medical services providers can help breastfeeding happen in the first place, and breastfeeding, in turn, becomes part of their job security. This mutual construction of breastfeeding and institutional authority starts to leak when breastfeeders violate any of the spoken or unspoken social norms or institutional rules in order to breastfeed—in effect, when their breastfeeding becomes "exceptional."

The writer Adrienne Rich declared that motherhood is an institution that is worthy of feminist suspicion and distinguishable from the loving act of mothering.[13] Inclusive language is hard to come by when talking about those who enact mothering but who do not identify with the gendered noun *mother*. This book includes many individuals such as gay fathers and transmasculine or nonbinary parents who take on primary roles in child-rearing, including nursing and breastfeeding. Barbara Katz Rothman makes the case that the verb "to mother" can be used to apply to anyone who does the work, regardless of their gender identity.[14] And so I use *mother* generally at times to avoid saying *others*, which is too cold (and, well, *othering*—as in exoticizing or marginalizing). Just *parents*, in everyday English, can apply to less participatory partners. *Breastfeeders* sounds too instrumental, but I use it reluctantly for lack of a better word.[15]

Exceptional breastfeeders have to make their way through a thicket of external blame and self-doubt just to do the mundane work of nourishing their babies. They may suddenly find themselves at the vanguard, confronting and reshaping core Western values like individual choice, scientific authority, and gender essentialism. They may not look much like the quintessential Madonna-and-baby dyad with their breast pumps and external feeding devices attached at the chest. But they do intense moral work at the boundaries of what society deems acceptable, defending and even promoting their alternative ways of breastfeeding.

By examining "others' milk" from these edges—and looking into the interstices of what gets considered "normal" breastfeeding—we can glimpse ordinary life that is also exceptional, extraordinary, and always political.

GOING WITH THE FLOW: THE SOCIAL CONTEXTS OF BREASTFEEDING

Breastfeeding is in the midst of a decades-long comeback. My mother likes to point out that when I was born in 1972, everyone told her that it was too hard and not worth the effort. That year marks the lowest breastfeeding initiation rate (22 percent) in U.S. history.[16] But by the time my brother was born in 1975, the now-international, probreastfeeding organization of women—originally a group of Catholic, well-to-do, stay-at-home mothers from Illinois—known as La Leche League (LLL or "La Leche") had succeeded in making its case more widely known.[17] My mom was able to breastfeed my brother with no problems for six weeks, a duration that was typical at that time. (Today, more than 81 percent of U.S. women initiate breastfeeding, and about half of all birthing women continue for at least six *months*.[18]) When La Leche formed in the 1950s, it was the atomic age, a regime of social progress and science during which the promise of medicine seemed to know no bounds. Doctor-approved—and hospital-promoted—formulations, engineered by expert chemists to contain a precise measure of vitamins and healthful chemicals was ideologically preferable to mother's milk,[19] a substance that could not (yet) be packaged and sold at the grocery store. People trusted science and business but not women. Instead, men of science and politicians, the benefactors of science, worked to thoroughly manage and monitor women's bodies. Obstetric interventions routinely put women into "twilight sleep," only to have them come to after it was over, remembering nothing of their babies' births.[20] And of course, women had too little control of their own procreative futures. Abortion, still under constant threat, was outright illegal from the nineteenth century, when worries about well-off whites' low birth rates took hold, to 1973, when its status changed with *Roe vs. Wade.*

Women pushed back, and La Leche's message rose along with the second-wave women's movement, which was at full crest by the mid-1970s.

The breastfeeding rate rose to 62 percent by 1982 partly due to LLL's influence. Its popular how-to guide titled *The Womanly Art of Breastfeeding* is still a standard. Feminists and environmentalists, as historian Jacqueline H. Wolf shows,[21] also worked concertedly toward changing public attitudes about breastfeeding. They emphasized breastfeeding as natural and the purview of women, not paternalistic doctors. This view happened to fit in well with the "earth mother" ideal popularized by hippies. (A different strain of feminists viewed motherhood as a trap, and they refused to accept what they saw as a deterministic and essentialist idea that women are meant to be mothers.[22])

The 1977 Nestle boycott helped spread the breastfeeding message. Activists decried the company's formula marketing tactics in the less industrialized parts of the world, where parents had no choice but to mix the stuff with contaminated water, a practice that led to infant deaths. They also criticized the company's collusion with hospitals, which passed out free formula in the industrialized West. This protest spanned the wealthy parts of the globe—including Canada, the United Kingdom, New Zealand, Australia, the United States, France, Sweden, and Germany—and led to the World Health Organization's (WHO) rules about breastfeeding standards and infant formula promotion.[23]

It is no coincidence that my mom got divorced at the same time that divorce rates skyrocketed. C. Wright Mills offers the concept of the *sociological imagination*, which means that what seem like individual circumstances resulting from an array of personal decisions are, in actuality, strongly shaped by social forces.[24] My mother wore long hair and bell-bottoms back then because those too were the trends. And the legal codification of no-fault divorce and concomitant shifts in social mores meant that she could also be a single mother and face less stigma. Soon she could have it all: the era of the "working mom" coincided with her second marriage and new career opportunities. (It seems that society forgot that all mothers work and that poor women and women of color have always worked for others.)

When the 1980s arrived, gone were my mother's avocado-green and harvest-gold appliances, her macramé plant hangers, and her sexy secretary persona. She had appeared as "Miss Utilities Management" in a newspaper photo series during the energy crisis 1970s. It included cheesecake shots of her in a miniskirt and a bikini as she conserved energy by turning out lights and watering the lawn only in the evening. Now with coiffed hair and shoulder-padded suit jackets, she became a "personnel officer"—today, a "human resources manager"—who could bring home the bacon and fry it up in a pan. Her own breastfeeding days were past, but her colleagues working nine to five now had to pull off intensive motherhood while also keeping up with men in the workplace.

This tense milieu is probably the origin of what Rothman calls mothers-as-fathers.[25] Middle-class, professional mothers of the eighties exaggerated their shoulders to look more like men; they had to be tough and less feminine. I always think of the actress Melanie Griffith's character in the Hollywood blockbuster *Working Girl*; she gets a short haircut the instant she goes from a secretary who is not taken seriously to a no-nonsense, successful businesswoman. *Her* secretary (Joan Cusack) continues to represent the other option as she offers suggestively to a visiting executive (Harrison Ford), "Coffee? Tea? [pause] Me?" Either way, there was no room for motherhood in the workplace—school-aged kids were home alone for hours between the bus drop off and the end of the workday—and there were few rooms, if any, set aside for pumping breast milk.

Yet babies and milk-producing bodies refused to comply with typical work hours invented for men by men. There were a couple of fixes, however. Technological improvements to breast pumps, from the 1980s until now, allowed women to relieve engorgement during a long day at work and still keep up with their careers. Mothers could be more like what fathers were thought to be, coming home from work at the end of the day to dispense advice and help with homework, spending weekends amassing quality time. The daily work of raising little ones could be outsourced to a veritable village of low-paid day care providers, tutors, and coaches.[26] Rothman observes, "Life seems to be switching from production to consumption."[27]

By the 1990s, another cruel twist emerged. Professional women were expected to also somehow perform an all-consuming dedication to their children. Sociologist Sharon Hays calls this ideology *intensive mothering*.[28] Even while outsourcing care, everyone expected mothers to be fully responsible for their children's health, happiness, and behavior. This expectation has not gone away. Mothers' tasks include monitoring every morsel of food, personally watching out for every possible danger, preventing any potential emotional trauma, ensuring that their children are constantly entertained and enriched, and immersing themselves in their children's education. Gone are the latchkey kids of Generation X. *Concerted cultivation* is the current middle-class standard.[29] As a society, we believe that parents need to carefully shape their children for their future as productive and successful citizens. This standard sets the bar impossibly high for everyone, but it is especially out of reach for poorer families, who lack the required cultural and economic capital to even approximate the ideal.

Mothers find that they cannot quite achieve the quantity or the quality of time they want with their families; they are tired from work and the "second shift"—the cooking, cleaning, household management, and childcare that still fall disproportionately on mothers.[30] Add nighttime breastfeeding, and you have chronic lack of sleep too.[31] Even college-educated, white mothers, who would seem to enjoy the most privileges and the most freedom, feel squeezed between motherhood and career. In trying to perform as ideal mothers, they struggle to also be the fulfilled individuals and prosperous consumers that society expects of them.[32] (Attachment parenting is one popular, intensive child-rearing philosophy that requires constant physical contact, from baby wearing to cosleeping, which can be very difficult to sustain.) There are identity-laden decisions at every turn: stay at home or work full time? Vaccinate or forgo the shots? Homeschool or send to public school? Breastfeed around the clock or give bottles of formula? No matter what you do, you are wrong.

STRATIFIED BREASTFEEDING

Of course, all of these are the options of the privileged. There are plenty of women who must work to survive and yet find themselves at the mercy of itinerant employment as they try to juggle work and childcare.[33] These parents cannot escape the scrutiny of authority. Poor women, for instance, cannot easily stay home, simply decide to refuse vaccines, or keep their children out of school. Child Protective Services (CPS), truancy officers, and welfare officials are watching. Using case studies of breast-feeders caught up in the CPS system, Jennifer Reich examines "the complex and contradictory ways that breastfeeding signals maternal commitment and danger."[34] Judges and social workers, she shows, may understand breast-feeding as dedicated mothering or as immoral, incompetent, and even abusively exposing their infants to drugs and pathogens. The authorities' preexisting biases seem to determine which view they end up taking.

The mommy wars, intensified by media stories, snarky memes, and internet trolls, constrain options, drawing and redrawing boundaries around acceptable mainstream motherhood. An internet meme reads, "I'm not a crunchy mom. I'm not a tiger mom. I'm not a free-range mom. I'm not a soccer mom. I'm not an attachment mom. I'm just a regular mom trying not to raise assholes." Some parents frame vaccination refusal as a consumer right; the pediatrician is not an authority but a service provider, and the baby's parents are the customers.[35] For others, bottle-feeding is a fine choice, and militant "lactivists" (lactation activists)—in poorly sketched caricature—are trying to pry women out of the workforce and keep them at home where they belong.[36] Some portray homeschoolers as religious zealots raising kids who will not be able to interact socially. Like many wars, these skirmishes that seem so ideologically opposed amount to border disputes. Although there are extreme outliers, there are vast middles with much in common. Some just want to delay vaccinations—they do not oppose all biomedicine in theory. Many need to mix-feed their babies with both bottle and breast in order to manage their busy lives. Some bypass failing schools by forming high-quality homeschool collectives with local experts teaching various subjects. For all their infighting, these seemingly disparate groups share an investment with the basic outlines of intensive mothering, with all its assumptions about femininity, consumer choice, family form, capitalism, and individualism.[37] The squabbles emanate from the same dominant social positions, from groups who share the same core values and who draw from the same "cultural logics" of intensive mothering.[38] Researchers find that breastfeeders and formula feeders both rely on themes of health, convenience, economy, and bonding to uphold their infant feeding choices.[39] Indeed, any feeding style can require around-the-clock mothering labor, which, by being self-sacrificing, conforms to the ideology of intensive mothering.

This ideology provokes ever more sanctimonious portrayals of bad mothers, however. The legal system perpetuates the bias that poor women lack the judgment to be good mothers. There are news stories about struggling single mothers getting arrested for leaving their children alone at home or in parked cars—however briefly—while they run out for groceries or interview for a job. By contrast, some middle-class professionals who practice "free-range" parenting—an intentional practice of less supervision for the purpose of nurturing the children's autonomy—can defend themselves by speaking out in the media or by obtaining attorneys to argue for their individual rights as parents. Jennifer Reich, who happened to be breastfeeding during the time of her CPS study, draws a sharp contrast between how members of the court system negatively judged poor women's breastfeeding while they actively accommodated Reich's own need to pump when she was at work in court environments.[40] Worse persecution comes in the form of arrests and prosecution of bereaved parents who watered down baby formula (called "formula stretching") without realizing that it could lead to fatal brain swelling. News stories make these parents into public examples, less to educate everyone about the dangers of giving babies water, perhaps, and more to delineate the good parents from the bad.

Stratified reproduction—the entrenched, systematic practice that commends the parenthood of the upper echelons of society while treating the procreation of lower status groups as a problem[41]—extends to infant-feeding practices. Breastfeeding and all its paraphernalia now serve as markers of class distinction, with formula cans and baby bottles cast as passé or even visible evidence of parenting failure.

Women of color, lesbians, gender nonconforming parents, parents with lower socioeconomic status, and other minorities—in effect, those who tend to find their personal biographies drawn outside the established boundaries—negotiate additional struggles with parenting and with breastfeeding. "Free the nipple!" some women declare at nurse-ins in airport terminals or in front of businesses after an episode of shaming has gone viral. The uneasy decision to breastfeed in public redoubles for women from religious backgrounds that emphasize modesty (such as Mormons and Muslims) and for masculine-identified breastfeeding parents. Devin, a queer gestational parent of one child, explained:

> Depending on the situation, I want to cover up because I don't want to satisfy anyone's prurient interest in this butch, this masculine person breastfeeding. Exposing her breast and putting a baby up to it. . . . I think the potential for people to be weirder, [thinking] "this isn't a normal heterosexual person in a married relationship doing what comes natural to her body; this is a some sort of queer freak feeding her kid." Mostly when I'm in public, like I'm in a restaurant and I'm someplace where I want to relax and enjoy myself—I don't feel like dealing with anyone. So I feel like covering up, and that's just totally

different. In general, I've gotten less confrontational in my life. In general, I'm like a fuck-you-I-do-what-I-want kind of person and so that's a change for me. There's a way that I feel like it is none of your fucking business what my boob looks like. I guess I could consider a different strategy were anything to happen, confront it head-on. I just don't have the energy for that.

Devin refused to be a spectacle. Before the baby arrives, their[42] masculine appearance plus swollen belly occasionally garnered some looks and odd behavior from people in coffee shops and other places—one woman's hostile, head-swiveling stare was particularly unnerving. But when it comes to nursing, Devin felt too exhausted from all the work of child rearing, plus all the work of their paid job, to deal with strangers' ignorance on top of it all.

Pivot to a different intersection: black women in the South who I interviewed sometimes had to face off with their own well-meaning mothers and mothers-in-law—an awkward prospect if these grandmothers happen to be providing the bulk of the childcare—who continued to give bottles of formula on the sly, thereby undermining the mother's wishes and milk supply.[43]

For their part, low-income mothers receiving financial help from the Women, Infants, and Children Food and Nutrition Service (WIC) must attend breastfeeding seminars to encourage that feeding choice. Yet it can be impossible to hold down a punch-the-clock job while attending to the need to either nurse their babies or pump their milk.[44] They have to supplement with formula, which may contribute to dwindling milk production and, sometimes, to increasing feelings of guilt and inadequacy. Sociologist Joan Wolf offers the term *total motherhood* to describe this demand for utter dedication of mother's bodies to wholly eliminating any and all risks to their babies.[45]

Society now considers breastfeeding the responsible feeding choice. One public health campaign to promote breastfeeding warned, "A healthy baby begins with you,"[46] and a baby-products retailer went with the slightly more ominous admonition, "His well being depends on you."[47] There is a widespread notion that formula is inferior and even "yucky" and potentially dangerous and that human milk is morally and nutritionally pure and wholesome and can even bump up baby's IQ.[48]

There may be an expectation to breastfeed, but those who do so experience insults to their efforts at every turn. The overarching grassroots message on the dozens of breastfeeding and milk-sharing blogs and Facebook groups? Breastfeeding is a right worth fighting for. The moderators of Black Women Do Breastfeed (BWDBF), which has more than 168,000 followers at the time of this writing, post images on Facebook of black women breastfeeding in an effort to normalize this choice. Black women in the United States are the least likely to breastfeed for a number of reasons.[49] First, slavery treated black women as chattel, valued mainly for their reproduction and for their work as wet nurses (for white women's babies and for other enslaved women's babies).[50] By the twentieth century, society cast them as foils to hygienic and progressive "scientific motherhood." Black and brown women and poor women, mischaracterized as closer to nature, were the only ones who lowered themselves to breastfeed in this view. And then, eventually, black women were excluded from the women's movement in which many white women reclaimed breastfeeding.[51] I've noticed that when black women post pictures of themselves breastfeeding, one common response from trolls, skeptical other women, and men is that they are flaunting themselves to get attention. One volunteer moderator mentioned to me that her team spends countless hours removing these sorts of negative posts to maintain an encouraging space.

With all of the advocacy for normalizing breastfeeding—as if it is not yet the norm—it might be surprising to realize that powerful institutions already aggressively promote it. WIC wants women to breastfeed; it is cheaper than providing formula.[52] Hospitals are increasingly "baby-friendly"—if not always mother-friendly—in that they curtail the formula-pushing that is known to impair attempts at breastfeeding and they provide lactation consultants to help their patients get started.[53] The Affordable Care Act required insurance companies to pay for breast pumps. This move served to keep women at work and, simultaneously, the argument goes, to keep babies healthier and therefore less of a draw on public resources. What, then, is the problem? Why does breastfeeding continue to be so fraught? And how can the study of exceptional breastfeeding help answer these questions?

AN OTHER-FRIENDLY INITIATIVE:
PRODUCING MILK, PRODUCING KNOWLEDGE

A classic quote by novelist David Foster Wallace says that fish don't know they are in water. So it goes for people immersed in the mainstream of breastfeeding. Those on the periphery of a social group, though, are highly aware of their differences—sometimes painfully so. It becomes easier for them to notice what the in-group takes for granted. Black feminist thinkers like bell hooks and Patricia Hill Collins show that centering on the experiences of those who are marginalized by society reveals the hidden rules, the mechanisms of social hierarchies, and the counterphenomena of resistance.[54] I interviewed breastfeeders whose practices they themselves deemed exceptional; I did so with the hope of tapping into some of the wisdom and insights being generated at the margins.

I began this study by interviewing eighty-three exceptional breastfeeders. I found them by word-of-mouth referrals and with an email that went almost viral. I messaged a friend, asking if she knew of any people who might be interested in talking with me about their "nonnormative" breastfeeding experiences; she forwarded this note to her contacts in a local birth doula group. Hundreds of responses flooded my inbox, coming from all over the United States as well as a few from Canada, the United Kingdom, Australia, and New Zealand. Several of these correspondents participated in semistructured, in-depth interviews with me—in person when feasible, over online video chats, or on the phone. I also interviewed a few exceptional breastfeeders from my personal networks. The initial interviews lasted between one and two hours, and I followed up with several of them with additional clarifying questions over email, social media, and telephone. So-called snowball sampling, in which respondents recommended other participants, helped me find several breastfeeders from a range of demographic groups (see appendix). With one exception,[55] all names (some chosen by the respondents themselves) and various identifying details have been changed to protect their privacy.

I also followed the posts of numerous public Facebook groups, Twitter feeds, and breastfeeding-related websites including but not limited to Breastfeeding USA, Breastfeeding MAFIA, Breastfeeding Mama Talk, Milk Junkies, Kelly Mom, Scary Mommy, The Leaky Boob, BWDBF, The Milk Meg, The Badass Breastfeeder, Eats on Feets (a riff on the Meals on Wheels charity), Occupy Breastfeeding, and Human Milk for Human Babies (HM4HB) from August 2014 to April 2017.[56] I systematically sampled comments from three Facebook groups (BWDBF, Eats on Feets, and HM4HB[57]) to get an idea of the patterns of the online interactions, and I also collected ad hoc screenshots of particularly relevant or unusual discussions. I use some of these posts to illustrate certain ideas throughout this book. My method does not call for random sample–generating techniques because the point here is not to precisely document the prevalence or likelihood of breastfeeding behaviors in any generalizable way but rather to understand why someone may engage in exceptional breastfeeding and to glean the range of meanings that these situations generate. I want to know *their* reasons (rather than my guesses) for engaging in these practices given the many obstacles and social costs involved. Again, to protect the identities of the commenters in various threads, I deliberately obscure the origins of many posts in order to limit the online searchability.

I observed several free breastfeeding classes that took place at two California hospitals and were led by three different lactation consultants. One of the groups wound up in a public protest when a beloved lactation consultant was suddenly fired; I attended the rally and asked questions informally, explaining my role as a researcher.[58] This book also includes some autoethnographic elements—I mine some of the insights I gained as an exceptional breastfeeder myself. My position as both an insider and an outsider trying to understand others' experiences obviously affects my research from recruiting participants to forming conclusions. For example, when I confessed that I had breastfed my soon-to-be adoptive son when he was still technically in foster care, one previously reticent respondent, Margaret, let loose with many secrets of her own. Several (but not all) asked me whether I breastfed; one person waited until the end of the interview, and when I answered in the affirmative, she said triumphantly, "I knew it!" My line of questioning likely gave it away.

My understanding also gets filtered through my own lens as a white, middle-class, feminist sociologist and anthropologist. What interview respondents told me were the stories they wanted me to hear, based, in part, on who I am to them. My conversation with Ameena Ali, PhD, a midwife and activist-scholar in the Afrocentric home birth and "blacktivist" (black lactation activist) movement, exemplifies how we together produce *situated knowledge*.[59] After telling me about her work and her philosophy of making home birthing and breastfeeding options available and affordable to more women of color—regardless of their status regarding incarceration, HIV, or employment—she stopped herself and quizzed me on my intentions: "When I hear that people are asking questions about community involvement, I really want to know what their purpose is. But I really want to hear from *you* [original emphasis]. Anybody can put things on paper, but I really want to hear what your passions are, and that helps me know how to market [my position]."

Perhaps assured that my motives aligned sufficiently with hers, she remarked (kindly, I should add), "Maybe what I'm saying is not something that is being respected; my words are not being heard. Maybe that you are saying the exact same thing that I've been saying for fifteen years, maybe someone will listen." Dr. Ali's remarks make it clear that she recognized my privilege and my views as a white academic. Can there be any doubt that *my* attempts to represent her position and her experience will fall short in capturing *her* full meaning and experience?

Sociologist Judith Stacey once asked, "Can there be a feminist ethnography?"—to which her answer was a qualified no.[60] There are always some elements of misinterpretation, some exploitation of less privileged others. The onus is on ethnographers to both recognize that they are never all-knowing scientists doing no harm and mitigate the damage to the extent that it is possible to do so. How can researchers minimize our intrusiveness in others' lives and keep from exploiting and even bastardizing their innermost thoughts and experiences for our own ends as scholars? For me, owning my biases and shortcomings, laying bare my own life, and acknowledging my various privileges are necessary steps. At the very least, the reader can come to a conclusion about how much credence to give the work and its conclusions. I include my own experiences to join in the resistance against restrictions to breastfeeding.

I try to demonstrate respect by believing the people I interviewed and observed and by attempting to tell their stories faithfully.[61] An op-ed piece appearing in *The Root* illustrates my point: the author decries the medical establishment for dismissing black women's self-reports of pain from endometriosis and accuses them of committing "therapeutic nihilism" (accepting the disease as a given outcome) instead of offering care.[62] I take this as a lesson that when doctors, or researchers of any stripe, think they know best, they invalidate people's lives.

One could approach a study of breastfeeding like this: probreastfeeding slogans such as "Until one, food is just for fun" (referring to the notion that breast milk alone provides sufficient nutrients for the first twelve months of life) not only reflect a 180-degree change from preferring science-backed formula to mother's milk but also reveal that we as a society value female bodies for their reproduction even to the detriment of a woman's autonomy. She may not be able to readily succeed in her career *and* breastfeed exclusively until age one. The pressure is put on individual mothers and their bodies to ensure that their babies get the "best," since the best is clearly what we as a society value. I could trace the nineteenth-century origins of the cult of true womanhood, in which being a mother was the ultimate expression of white women's femininity, and the contemporaneous construction of children as precious.[63] And then I could go on to examine the evolution of Enlightenment ideas about individualism. At a certain point, though, the study of what breastfeeding *represents* reiterates what we already understand about social forces and blurs the importance of real, meaningful experiences. Feminist scholars who study science note that social researchers in the late twentieth and early twenty-first centuries have been so focused on deconstructing and interpreting the meanings of things that we sometimes forget about on-the-ground experiences.[64]

There is plenty of merit in digging around for inherent meanings—tracing the development of naturalized ideas and critiquing these assumptions are vitally important. For example, one proposed breastfeeding campaign created for a pediatric society in Sao Paolo, Brazil, depicts babies at their mothers' breasts, but the breasts are a doughnut with sprinkles, a soda, or a greasy cheeseburger. The slogan admonishes, "Your child is what you eat."[65] Apparently, the contractor decided not to launch the campaign due to a strong media backlash against its method of shaming mothers who would eat unhealthy foods. This ad is just an extreme instance of the kinds of representations about breastfeeding, mothers, and women that infiltrate Western society, from signs and slogans to hospital pamphlets, media stories, blogs, and websites. Scholars can identify our beliefs about who should be breastfeeding and how it should be done through this sort of investigation. As anthropologist and sociologist Bruno Latour points out, beliefs are not mental states; they are all about social relations.[66] Breastfeeding not only reflects and responds to social forces but also is active in creating social forces.

If I am to centralize the problems of exceptional breastfeeders, I have to admit that breastfeeding is more than the sum of its parts. To explain, there is a difference between describing breastfeeding and doing it. Breastfeeding is a process, an identity, and a performance. Breastfeeding is a relationship. Breastfeeding is social. Breastfeeding is both nutritive and nurturing. Breastfeeding is emotional. Breastfeeding is natural and mammalian and physiological. Breastfeeding is also malleable; psychological trauma and stress can stop the flow of milk, and yet, conversely, breastfeeding can calm a stressed system. It makes for intangible feelings and relations. The experience of bonding during breastfeeding involves the exchange of warmth and the production of physiological and emotional sensations. The entangled *intra-actions* (to borrow Karen Barad's dense concept)[67] of a baby's and a mother's bodily processes, their mutual comfort and love, and, importantly, their social relations produce bonding. Bonding is a particularly diffuse abstraction that parents rarely question but that everyone agrees is vitally important. Psychologists operationalize it as "attachment," with attachment disorders resulting from improper or insufficient nurturing in infancy. But bonding also connotes a bioemotional state and mental status that each person experiences differently.

Performing bonding makes it real. Even as a feminist observer wary of any essentialist proclamations about women's bodies, I cannot doubt that these feelings exist. But I can question any sneaking assumption that breastfeeding is the only way, or even the superior way, to make these deep connections.

The breastfeeding relationship is constantly emerging, and this is why the concept of *intra-actions* is more accurate than *interactions*. It is not the result of two or more individuals interacting with one another; instead the participants create each other's roles and relations. Lanie, a mother of six, described how she came to know the meaning of breastfeeding: "I really believe that breastfeeding is best. I now believe that that can look like a lot of different things and best doesn't necessarily just mean from nipple to the baby's mouth. It can be different things and still be best. I get a really huge feeling of love inside me, a surge, happiness inside, and just feeling so connected, like, it just feels like beauty. The word 'beauty' means something more than pretty. It would be—this is probably silly, right? It feels beautiful and warm and loving and connected and perfect. I love it. I love it." Lanie referred to subjective sentiments like *love, happiness, connection,* and *beauty*.

She equated breastfeeding to all sorts of wonderful things even as she utterly dismantled the common definition of breastfeeding. There is more to breastfeeding, and to all phenomena, than what we can measure and describe. Introducing flexibility and invoking the sacred in procreative matters, as Lanie did, disrupt linear, medically and scientifically circumscribed assumptions. Wendy Simonds shows how the "spiritual" aspects of skilled home birth midwifery challenge the medical preoccupation with isolating and then timing each component of the birth process.[68] And Alison Bartlett expands on Simonds' work to argue that a mystical experience of breastfeeding similarly allows for "alternative scenarios" that decenter biomedicine.[69] Nature, culture, and the meanings we construct cannot adequately be studied as separate things.

Breastfeeding is always mediated through social relationships, biology, and social forces. As Barbara Katz Rothman says about birth, "There is no 'natural' for us to compare."[70] Katherine A. Dettwyler compares breastfeeding in a handful of non-Western cultures to drive home this point.[71] In Mali, breasts have no sexual meaning whatsoever and are considered to be just for breastfeeding babies. Among the Mende people of Sierra Leone, because sex with men during breastfeeding is blamed for nursing infants' malnutrition, weaning happens much earlier. The meaning of breasts and breastfeeding varies across cultures, within different social groups, and throughout history. However, it is a universal fact that humans have a very hard time learning to breastfeed (and to have the time and support to continue breastfeeding) without help from others, and, of course, the caregiving breastfeeder's and the baby's bodies must cooperate.

It would be wrong for me to say that what a breastfeeder thinks she does is not what she really does. When an exclusive pumper, someone who pumps all her milk and gives it to the baby in a bottle, for instance, tells me that she "breastfed" for a year, then that is what she has done. In making an effort to listen and to keep from reflexively reinterpreting what she "really" means, I am trying to refrain from erasing her experience. Still, as ethnographer Kath Ryan and her team argue, the intimacy lost should be a cause for concern.[72] Pumping milk as a matter of routine eases the way toward more commodification and commercialization of breast milk. Two or more logically opposed ideas might exist at the same time. Some exclusive pumpers may insist that they are breastfeeding precisely as a counterclaim against others' concerns about the quality of their intimacy.

Brazilian anthropologist Eduardo Viveiros de Castro suggests that perhaps we are all anthropologists (including breastfeeders themselves in this case) and that scholars should be wary of "giving reasons for the natives' reasons."[73] Vanessa, a mother of three, related a harrowing story of her adoptive daughter's time in an orphanage and then an abusive foster home. The traumatized child, once placed with Vanessa's family, suffered from lack of sleep, and she could not calm down, disliking any touch. Eventually, at age five, she asked to breastfeed and, around the same time, Vanessa happened upon a heartfelt essay from someone in a similar situation. This other woman's story, and Vanessa's desperate need to soothe the child, led her to acquiesce: "She would actually wake distressed, she'd actually breastfeed, and then she would fall asleep again. And it was just like magic. It was amazing. I hadn't necessarily expected that that would happen. And I hadn't actually known whether it would be something that would be possible to do."

Some advocates and researchers express particular discomfort with breastfeeding and breast milk being called magic or magical, possibly because they worry that this property is unscientific or that imbuing it with such power will make parents who use formula feel inadequate.[74] One could argue that Vanessa is using "magic" figuratively here, and she is. Yet almost all the breastfeeders I talked with and observed spent some time marveling at the magic of milk and breastfeeding. We can choose to take their words at face value, to stay open to the concept of magic—in whatever meaning it has for them—to avoid the impulse to explain it away. Anthropologist Anna Tsing proposes the concept of *productive misunderstandings*—differences between local knowledge (in this case, magic) and that of the ethnographer (who might not believe in magic) that can produce helpful insights (breastfeeding means more than nutrition and comfort for the baby).[75] Multiplying ideas is more productive than reducing them.

And yet this very idea of magic does not originate solely from caregivers' grounded experience. Magic can be co-opted—unwittingly or with premeditation—and sold back to caregivers with dubious results. Biological anthropologist Katie Hinde points out the sexist pattern in which the science of breastfeeding and breast milk lags behind studies that interest men, like, say, erectile dysfunction, which receives ample funding support.[76] As a result of this uneven funding, too little is known about what exactly composes breast milk and how it varies depending on the physiology of breastfeeder and baby. Advocates who cite this frontier research strive to "unravel the mystery of human milk."[77] It is so inscrutable to be almost magical, a patronizing view of women's bodies. It is like Edward Said's critical notion of *orientalism*, in which Westerners assume that Eastern cultures are impossibly exotic.[78]

Formula companies market this magic. For example, they have seized upon the findings of small studies that suggest a health benefit of a chemical compound (a particular oligosaccharide, of which there are many) found in breast milk.[79] They then produced this chemical into a packaged powder that loving parents can sprinkle and mix into formula—ostensibly, to make it more like breast milk. Similac's Pro-Advance infant formula sports the paradoxical label "HMO Human Milk Oligosaccharide" with an asterisk; in smaller print below, it reads "not from human milk." Researchers doubt that there are any benefits to this powder and even wonder if separating one chemical from the rest could actually be harmful.[80] But they do not yet have a full grasp on what components constitute breast milk, so it is hard to say. In one way of thinking, breast milk and breastfeeding demand closer scientific scrutiny to prevent a potential public health disaster, to give equal attention to female biology, and to better understand infant development. But the breathless reporting of each purported new benefit of breast milk begins to traffic in essentialism.[81] The exceptional breastfeeders I talked to often refer to "lots of research" that supports the aphoristic "breast is best" ideal.

Anthropologists who study magic across cultures find that people share a near-universal tendency to rely on it when outcomes are uncertain—like praying only in a crisis.[82] In a world that demands intensive mothering and concerted cultivation, every decision is on shaky ground, and each child's well-being is at stake. The science and magic of breastfeeding and breast milk become intertwined in such a way that exceptional breastfeeders go to plenty of trouble to do it whether or not they can articulate exactly why it is best. It just is—for them.

I strive to convey the intentions and the problems of creative breastfeeders in a way that they would recognize. To me, that means assuming that there are layers to their experiences. Breastfeeding can be many *processes* at once: feeding a baby, comforting a child, administering vitamins and immunities, performing motherhood, providing a relaxing respite for the breastfeeder, engaging in bonding, or experiencing magic.[83] Breastfeeders produce, in their bodily practice, milk and knowledge and relationships.

And it is a different set of processes for everyone. As I think about how Vanessa and others squeeze themselves through the myriad tensions wrought by science and medicine and total motherhood,[84] I imagine that they come out on the other side embodying a range of ways to be.

This research led me to ask another question: How can we free ourselves from the essentialist, biologistic ideological booby traps that surround breastfeeding and begin to move toward a more supportive, less alienating, less judgmental, perhaps even more communal, experience of raising the next generation?

INTERRUPTING THE FLOW: MORALIZING AND MEDICALIZING BREASTFEEDING

On September 3, 2012, former New York City mayor Michael Bloomberg, following a trend enacted by a few other governments, like in nearby Massachusetts and Rhode Island, began a citywide program asking maternity wards to keep their infant formula locked away. The aim of "Latch On NYC" was to counteract the all too easy practice of administering formula to newborns in the hospital, a practice that many researchers, lactation professionals, and new mothers say sabotages breastfeeding. Getting breastfeeding started can be challenging, especially in a hospital context where many high intervention births require recovery time and where medical personnel constantly interrupt sleep.[85] It can be difficult in the best of circumstances as the newborn-caregiver dyad negotiates the right position and a comfortable, effective mouth-to-breast latch. Unsurprisingly, Bloomberg's efforts unleashed a backlash—but not from indignant formula companies that could no longer send new parents home with a bag of freebie formula (like drug pushers offering a taste to potential customers) and not from detached nurses eager to stick a bottle in babies' mouths and get on with their tasks. The loudest protests came from women refusing to yield any more power over their bodies and their self-determination to external authorities. Commentators sometimes took a libertarian bent, in which they were aghast at the nerve of "the nanny state" government to tell people what to do; the reaction was similar to the attempts to ban large sugary drinks in New York City recently. But for some birthing women, the insult was less of an abstraction and more of a personal attack on their suitability for motherhood.

Politicians have a way of making female procreative bodies their business, from passing laws to restrict abortion access and funding for birth control to criminalizing miscarriage and stillbirth. The regulation and surveillance is never about making society a more livable place but about upholding moral positions, often by punishing the "sinners." Despite the fundamental belief that we are all individuals, the reality is that the most intimate aspects of our lives are under public scrutiny. The personal is political, and the private is public.

Who we are as private citizens, from our preferred romantic partners to our infant-feeding choices, becomes fodder for discussion in the public sphere, and that discussion then impacts our private behavior.[86] Yet at the same time, the legal philosophy of bodily integrity insists that individuals have the unassailable right to make any and all decisions regarding their own bodies.[87] The concept, if applied uniformly, would prevent forced sterilization, allow for uninhibited access to abortion and birth control, and allow "gender confirmation" surgery to those who choose to have it. Whether a person breastfeeds or not is clearly that person's own decision, even if authorities enact rules to discourage or to encourage the use of formula.

Breastfeeding and other aspects of child rearing involve more than one person's body. Bodily rights get into tricky territory when we consider whether parents can decline medical treatment for sick children or forgo vaccination. If immune-system-compromised individuals contract a deadly case of the measles because unvaccinated children spread the disease at Disneyland, can we hold their parents legally accountable, or is it the parents' right of bodily integrity by proxy not to risk vaccine injury? Is it their duty to protect their own children however they see fit?[88] Where do we draw the line about what rights parents have to interpret their children's health needs? As a society, we usually draw the line at violence. Could withholding treatments or vaccines be considered violence as a form of child abuse? Is it abusive to give children large sugary drinks?

Breastfeeding is a civic duty, as seen in one nonprofit's informational poster.[89] It includes "fewer sick days" and "lower health care costs" in a list of breastfeeding's many benefits, an ideological trend already noted by Glenda Wall in her deconstruction of Canadian breastfeeding pamphlets distributed by the state health care system.[90] Other advocates appeal to green consciousness by touting breastfeeding's lower environmental impact. Will formula-feeding parents be called to account for too many hospital visits

and too many sick days for their children's ear infections or diarrheal illnesses since some medical studies suggest breastfed babies have fewer of
these maladies? These parents are already in trouble for adding too much
water to the powder.

Can we accuse parents of turning out inadequate children if they skip
the "bonding" benefit by bottle-feeding pumped breast milk? Characters
in the final episode of the HBO series *Girls* seem to think as much. When
the protagonist, Hannah Horvath, has trouble breastfeeding, she blames
herself for her son's much-diminished future prospects.

Those who breastfeed feel unsupported and under attack from critics
who want to define how it is done as well as when, where, and for how long.
And those who formula-feed feel the sting of public scorn and, not rarely,
self-flagellation.[91] The question of breastfeeding is a "moral minefield" along
the transition to motherhood.[92]

Yet it does not even come down to two stark choices: breastfeed or not.
It is not entirely possible to even nail down a definition of breastfeeding.
Many parents "mix-feed" their infants, suckling at the breast and providing bottles of formula as needed. One lactation consultant and tandem
nursing (breastfeeding more than one child at a time) mother of three, Jessica, who herself encountered trouble with breastfeeding initially, told me
that her clients appreciate her as a "moderate." They thought of her this way
because she would suggest mixing strategies (and some parents literally mix
formula with breast milk in the same bottle) in order to keep some breastfeeding going rather than having someone give up altogether. Some mothers (including me) breastfeed one child and not the other for a wide range of
reasons like the baby's health, the mother's health, financial circumstances,
amount of support available at the time, and variations in milk production.

One need not even have female breasts; cisgender males and transmasculine fathers can "chestfeed" with or without having a nipple to suckle on.
I talked with some trans-identifying dads who have breasts but reimagine
and rename the activity (for some, their breasts are mechanistic components of a food-delivery system). Thomas, a cisgender gay dad, provided his
child with milk shipped by the baby's surrogate for an entire year across the
North American continent and an international border. He took turns with
his partner "breast milk feeding" with bottles of breast milk. While suckling at the breast is a "dynamic biological process" and "not just a meal at
the breast" as breast milk scientists show,[93] the closeness at the chest and

the perceived nutrition of the gestational mother's milk make Thomas's version "like-breastfeeding."

Still others do breastfeeding in different ways. A friend of mine helped inspire this research by cofeeding (sometimes called "cross nursing," "shared nursing," "allo-nursing" or "breastsharing") with another mother. Each mother left her child in the care of the other while she went to work, and the mother on baby duty changed the diapers, sang the lullabies, and nursed the hungry, fussy infants as needed. I interviewed several childcare providers with formal and informal "wet-nursing" arrangements. Babies get to nurse, and mothers can go to work or take care of other life business.

A variety of adaptive practices fall under the umbrella of "breastfeeding." One guileless commenter on HM4HB asked, "Isn't feeding your baby someone else's breast milk breastfeeding too?" Someone responded with an explanation that I have come to view as typical: "When I think of breastfeeding, I don't just think of latching at the breast and drawing out mom's milk. I think of feeding baby in any way that involves breast milk or the breast." The idea is to counter formula and/or bottles, to the degree possible, because these now symbolize a lack of maternal devotion.

Gestational mothers who exclusively pump—perhaps due to nipple shape, prohibitive work schedules, psychological and/or physical discomfort with breastfeeding due to a history of sexual abuse, or a baby's lack of appropriate sucking reflexes—often call what they are doing "breastfeeding." If the international boom in milk-sharing internet groups like HM4HB and Eats on Feets are any indication, a growing number of parents accept "informally"[94] donated milk on their children's behalf, giving human milk through a bottle or a supplemental nursing system (SNS). An SNS is a handy (once you get the hang of it) device that amounts to a bottle or bag of milk and/or formula hung around the neck with a tube leading to the nipple; the baby takes both nipple and tube into her mouth and not only receives nutrition and experiences closeness but may also stimulate milk production. A finger dripping milk or a small cup can work similarly. To many, all of these options constitute breastfeeding. A generous definition of breastfeeding is a form of solidarity that honors the parents' efforts to provide what they can. Calling all sorts of practices "breastfeeding" is also a declaration that one's caregiving conforms to the current standard.

Bottle-feeding breast milk is not an either/or proposition. Clearly the milk can come from more than one lactating individual; my first son received breast milk from seven of my friends and scores of anonymous (to me) donors who contributed to the nearby nonprofit milk bank. (The Mothers' Milk Bank of Santa Clara County operates on the grounds of a large regional hospital, but its funding comes from monetary donations and from selling the donor milk that they collect, test, and pasteurize. They get it from breastfeeders who they recruit from hospitals, medical providers' offices, and social media.) I like to attribute this early nutritional diversity to his current willingness to eat just about any food, and I even wonder if it accounts for his remarkable resistance to cold and flu viruses. We joked that the milk he received from an Australian coworker, who passed along what she pumped each day in the office, provided prophylactic protection from untold exotic illnesses like "kangaroo pox" and "wombat-borne diseases." The science that confirms breast milk's incredible properties contributes to this kind of magical thinking. Jeri and Allie, a same-gender, cofeeding couple who live in Los Angeles, laughed as Jeri said, "We want our baby to be superhuman." Allie amplified, "She's bionic. A little bionic baby!" These two moms also donated their freezer stash to other families with infants in order to share the wealth, saying that "it is good for them. . . . The more different types [of milk] they are introduced to, the better off their immune systems are."

Sami and Amelia, a couple who identify as lesbian, pushed the boundaries of breastfeeding just a bit more, further frustrating any attempts to operationalize, or precisely define, the concept. They both share genetic parentage of their child. Sami is a transwoman who briefly curtailed her feminizing hormone regimen to impregnate Amelia with her sperm. When Amelia went back to her paid job, Sami induced lactation. She used the Newman-Goldfarb protocol—a regimen of birth control pills and breast pumping developed by doctors for adoptive mothers—to help with breastfeeding. Both mothers also pumped their milk, and little Alex nursed with both mothers, calling out "Next one!" when he'd emptied a breast. At times, he had breast milk from bottles, particularly when visiting his grandparents.

Some lactation workers, parents, and researchers prefer the term *nursing* to *breastfeeding* as a catch-all that does not emphasize the nutritional aspect. But nursing also refers to a career and to all the intimate care we give to our sick loved ones. Once, my mother went with my infant son and me to a breastfeeding class. When we walked into the hospital building, she noticed a miniature marquee on a stand that read, "Nursing class." My mom noticed the arrow underneath that pointed to the right and started to head in that direction. But this was my second visit, and I remembered that the group I wanted was upstairs, not down the hall. The sign referred to a class for hospital nurses. A quick scan around the vestibule yielded a paper sign taped to the wall on which someone had written, "New moms' breastfeeding support, Second Floor."

The frequently used term *infant-feeding* is not adequate either. Sometimes a child will not begin breastfeeding, nursing, suckling, or chestfeeding until many months, even years, after being born. And suckling at the breast may yield little or no milk yet still deliver comfort to a child (and, often, to the breastfeeder). What exactly counts as breastfeeding varies by context and perspective. It may not matter all that much what we call the various infant-feeding choices. Perhaps we can start with the assumption that parents are doing the best that they can.

This plaintive, admittedly cliché proposal is immediately frustrated by the bald fact that powerful, faceless institutions and the engines of the media care precious little about harming women's self-concept or about increasing reproductive freedoms. They operate continually to preserve the status quo, and that can mean keeping groups in their place, from always denigrating the practices of poor women to ensuring that women's public struggles center on their bodies. It can be worrying to think about what might be next on the breastfeeding front: Courtney Jung's polemic *Lactivism*, a 2015 book critical of lactation activism, smacked of disdain for the one-dimensional, cultish proponents of breastfeeding advocacy that she encountered at Manhattan cocktail parties. I kept wondering if she was a harbinger of discerning women who could be becoming too sophisticated for breastfeeding. Jung recoils at the ostentatious class privilege on display in pricey breastfeeding-supply boutiques like Yummy Mummy, but perhaps the obsession with breastfeeding on the level of marking class identity is going the way of Lululemon yoga wear and Coach products: too accessible to the masses to retain its cachet. Might they return to wet-nursing nannies or begin purchasing breast milk on the consumer market? I imagine it on the grocery shelf, tastefully packaged, high-priced, sanitized, and dehumanized.

For now, though, consider that the pernicious maintenance of social hierarchies keeps the machine of capitalism running. Work schedules, and the internalization of the concept of productive work hours,[95] predestine breastfeeders to feel they have failed in one aspect or another: they must either give up their jobs to put their babies to breast on demand or resort to artificial means, utilizing pumps and bottles and risking exhaustion from nighttime feedings that can keep them from performing adequately at their jobs. Many researchers and advocates argue that babies are *supposed* to be up at night, but there is little hope that such a fact will budge the entrenched structure of the workweek.[96] The burden is on the breastfeeder.

Mika, a friend of mine, feels these burdens at home as well. She just had a baby, and like many American women, she feels very guilty for letting the house and the laundry and the niggling details of life slide into disarray as she breastfeeds seemingly all the time. Her predicament results from unrealistic standards for women, compounded by her anomic existence, cut off from the busy business of late capitalist life and from family who live a couple of states away. Yet she is no ideological dupe, tricked into believing what she does is the only morally correct way to behave; she knows full well that capitalist and patriarchal forces operate to isolate her and make her feel unproductive (even while she produces milk enough to grow a human) and that, at the same time, the social construction of motherhood contributes to her motivation to give the child all of herself lest he not get the best like any other kid is getting.

Her body is the site where these forces play out a game that Mika knows is not fair. Yet she also feels blissfully intoxicated by the experience of gazing at her baby, nursing him and humming lullabies in the cool, quiet night. Let us not forget the material reality produced and reproduced by warmth, heartbeats, nutrition, and hormones—the metaphysical, spiritually transporting experience that Mika describes (and that I have also experienced) and the mutual development of a close relationship. The context is not ideal, but she feels like breastfeeding is worth the effort.

Cricket's body was also the site of the power play of institutions: in particular, medicalization and one of its progeny: scientific motherhood. Cricket, a busy professional and mother to an athletic and sensitive nine-year-old girl she breastfed until age four, recalled pumping her breast milk: "What you do is watch the line. How much am I making? It is like you are competing with yourself. You have no control over it. It is not like you can make more. It is a scenario where you are disappointing yourself that you cannot make enough, that you can't control it. You have no power to create more. . . . It was just a chore. It was just a pain."

Here, unbiased tools, not intuition, produce the knowledge about what is going on with one's body. The self-competition reflects our culture's emphasis on individual success; we are always trying to win, and hitting goals extends to pumping milk and to breastfeeding in general. Marking breastfeeding duration and milk quantity can become obsessions. (One fastidious mother, who happens to be an accountant, told me she loved keeping track of the breastfeeding math with an app on her phone.) Cricket identified the source of her powerlessness and fought against her own urge to measure her production, but the tool she used—the graduated bottle with lines marking the ounces, much like a beaker from a high school chemistry class—made it impossible to avoid.

Medicalization, the inexorable process by which human conditions become subject to medical study and surveillance, especially applies to female procreative matters.[97] The menstrual cycle requires monitoring and remedies; a woman who does not get pregnant in due time, regardless of the reasons, is pathological; pregnancy is a disability; and births are medical emergencies. Or so it seems. Breastfeeding becomes a medical problem too—part of the overall clinical experience. Medicine, retaining its patriarchal foundations, is often more about furthering moral values than it is about healing illness.[98] Where doctors tend to want patient compliance, patients put their focus on getting their needs met.[99]

So when we want to understand why breastfeeding a foster child is illegal, aside from the rare judge's order, we can look to the potent mix of patriarchal, moralizing medicalization. The given reason for outlawing this type of nursing is that disease might be transmitted, though the breastfeeder could get cleared with blood tests and the milk itself can be tested. Similarly, clinics eliminate "gay" men[100] from blood donation opportunities in spite of the fact that anyone can pass on HIV and that the clinics test the blood anyway. There is a squeamishness about the body fluid that disguises the true objections: the desire to punish homosexuality and set it apart morally.[101] For breast milk, the moral objection stems from the ideological proscription against separating mother and baby (and, upsettingly, the unspoken—except by anonymous internet trolls—fear that sexual perversion might be going on).

Even though breast milk is food, medical perspectives will lump it in with all other potentially "dirty" body fluids.[102] One aghast lactation consultant told me that there was no way she would recommend any cofeeding arrangements due to what she says her profession calls "the ick factor"—many of her colleagues, I know, would disagree with this assessment. Yet these sorts of unscientific taboos infiltrate the experiences of breastfeeders, especially the unconventional, or "exceptional," ones I describe in this book.

Is breastfeeding a public health issue and not simply a lifestyle choice? The WHO, U.S. Surgeon General, Centers for Disease Control and Prevention (CDC), and American Academy of Pediatrics (AAP), many major hospitals, and other organizations say yes. Baby-friendly hospital initiatives (BFHIs), which have been around for twenty-five years, follow a "gold standard of care" that meets ten criteria, or steps to success, such as encouraging on-demand breastfeeding, forestalling any use of bottles and pacifiers, and educating patients and staff about the benefits of breastfeeding.[103] While lauded by many a breastfeeder who does not want to see her efforts undermined and who appreciates some help in getting it started, some of the steps can be rather unfriendly in practice. For example, part of the initiative requires that a lactation consultant visit within the hour of birth; beginning to breastfeed within this time frame has been shown to increase initiation rates. Some commenters on online breastfeeding support group threads lamented that immediately following emergency cesarean sections or other birth-related difficulties, they felt unready for the expert visit; then, later, when they became more alert, the lactation consultant was unavailable. The hospital fulfilled its objective by ticking off the item that calls for a lactation visit, but it did not actually enhance the woman's chances for breastfeeding. A few commenters online suggest that hospitals change their focus to being "mother-friendly" by instituting more flexible protocols. (Watch out, though: calls for "mother-friendly" regulations can be code for an attack on breastfeeding advocacy. *The Skeptical OB* blogger and provocateur Amy Tuteur writes sarcastically, "Apparently brain damaged and dead infants are a price that lactivists are willing pay to promote breastfeeding."[104] She dislikes BFHIs, denouncing them as based on pseudoscience. Tuteur thinks that advocates brainwash mothers to breastfeed even when their babies are starving and in need of formula supplementation.)

The big medical authorities on breastfeeding take an "evidence-based" approach that focuses on health outcomes in aggregate, which does not necessarily focus on individuals' optimal experience. But which outcomes should steer medical policy? Should the main concerns be the rate of breastfeeding initiation and its duration, or should breastfeeders' satisfaction figure in? Some mothers nurse on demand not just because hospital authorities advise it but also because scheduled feedings seem too clinical, too 1950s. But one study found that breastfeeders who stick to a schedule feel less stress and report less depression than the anytime, anywhere breastfeeders who are never off duty.[105] One breastfeeder, commenting online, questions the word "demand," which reminds her of more problematic "demands" on her body by others within rape culture—rampant sexually aggressive language and the trivialization of sexual assault.

So on which evidence will the policies be based? And for that matter, what aspects get studied to become evidence in the first place? Medicine has a history of going with whatever minimizes its costs and maximizes its control over women's supposedly unruly bodies.

Pathologization, an integral function of medicalization that seeks to find problems to fix, makes the everyday functions and cycles of female bodies into medical complications.[106] We all participate in this comprehensive strategy of control.[107] When Rhonda's baby kept spitting up, she told me in an interview, she immediately worried that there might be something seriously wrong. Did he have gastroesophageal reflux disease (GERD)? Was he getting sufficient nutrition? Was her milk bad in some way? Should she have done an elimination diet and stopped her dairy intake, her gluten intake? Other moms in her support group helped her consider all the possible problems. As a hypochondriac myself, I understand the neurotic worry; this is her *baby* we are talking about. Enter a wise and experienced lactation consultant. She finds out from Rhonda that her baby was gaining weight (check), that her baby did not cry when spitting up (check), and that her milk supply was quite robust (check). The diagnosis? Shrugging, the lactation consultant concludes, "So you have a laundry problem."

With the loss of a couple of generations of breastfeeding practice and the typical neolocal residence patterns (not so many of us still live near extended family once we grow up and have children), we have to rely on experts whose investments in medicalization vary. Resisting pathologization, one lactation consultant I observed leading a support group kept a wry smile on her face—which she dropped only to coo at babies—and calmed the anxious breastfeeders with pithy responses like, "Welcome to parenting, honey," "Every baby is different," "Do it however you want," and "Babies are resilient." It was clear to me that the lactation consultant had uttered these phrases too many times to count; the snappy delivery was assuring in its insouciance. She'd heard it all before. These parents' worries were normal, their breastfeeding challenges expected.

Scientific motherhood, borne of categorizing and measuring and identifying all observable phenomena, led to weighing babies, counting wet diapers, setting the clock for sleep times and feed times and tummy times.[108] It continues to prevail even among self-described "crunchy moms," who strive to eliminate any and all toxins and risks[109] from their babies' lives and to get back to a more natural way of mothering via cloth diapering, exclusive breastfeeding, cosleeping, and baby wearing.

Many breastfeeders find comfort and a sense of accomplishment in large freezer stashes of pumped milk—for instance, counting the number of bags and duly reporting the numbers on social media. (One of Susan Falls's milk-sharing interviewees called the freezer stash "emotional insurance"—a fitting description.)[110] I watched a room full of crunchy moms in a Northern California breastfeeding support group as each silently weighed her unclothed baby on the hospital-supplied scale, which occupied pride of place in the center of the room, immediately before and after nursing. Some repeated the ritual twice or more over the course of the ninety-minute session. They could not measure their milk by volume visually, but they could see the ounces tick upward on the scale and thus collect data to monitor their output scientifically. Much hangs in the balance: one clinical study found that weighing newborns to ascertain how much milk they were getting triggered feelings of "gratitude," "guilt," "disappointment," and "fear" in the breastfeeding mothers.[111]

It is in this context of the medicalized, scientific, moral authority within capitalism that breastfeeders experience their bodies and their relationships. Yet there is plenty of friction here with abundant opportunities for productive misunderstandings[112] and for subversion in the spaces between when breastfeeding goes as society expects and when it does not.

EXPRESSING SUPPORT: DECOLONIZING
AND QUEERING BREASTFEEDING

> My thought in my head is "I've got to get past that nine-month mark. I have to get past that nine-month mark, I have to." I do not know why. But all these moms there [at a hospital support group] were still nursing at eighteen months. And I'm like, "I can do that." I can do that because there's not a single [other] person in this group that's of color. I've got to do it. I didn't have anything to prove to anyone, and I wasn't trying to, but I was like nobody else in my community. No one knows about doulas and midwives and nursing. I don't want to put anyone in a box, but privileged women get to afford something like this. That's usually middle-class white women.
>
> —Imani

Breastfeeding poses challenges even in the most ideal circumstances. Popular imagination often assumes mothers to be avid consumers, not too young and not too old, white and middle class and married, adherents to Judeo-Christian values, and willingly subject to authority. If these descriptors held true for everyone, we might just be able to tackle any and all problems that emerge with breastfeeding. If the problem is mastitis, a common systemic infection caused by blocked milk ducts, why, just take some antibiotics, hire a housecleaner, and have your husband take off work for a week to take care of you! Follow the Mayo Clinic's advice and "review your breastfeeding technique with your doctor," who may suggest that you make an appointment with a lactation consultant.[113] Perhaps your mother-in-law thinks formula would be better so she can feed the baby too and so everyone can be sure the baby is getting enough food. Just hand her the WHO guidelines and the breastfeeding pamphlet from the pediatrician's office; those authorities will surely hold sway with her!

These sorts of solutions work better in bureaucrats' minds than in Imani's world. She is a single mother whose family gives her constant grief about breastfeeding because it seems immodest, show-offy, or even like she is pretending to be white. She and some other black women I talked with count their mothers' and their aunts' and their in-laws' eventual sighing, eye-rolling acquiescence as resounding successes because they know that is as much as they are going to get.

Imani's experience does not represent that of all black women, just as my experiences do not represent all white women. But our disparate experiences do provide a potent reminder of why we start feminist social research assuming the primacy of intersectionality.[114] This (now widely misunderstood and sometimes maligned)[115] perspective emanates from black feminist thought and says that everyone possesses a multiplicity of identities and social statuses and that each separately, and in combination, result in different life experiences and afford different access to privilege in a stratified society. As activist Audre Lorde said in a 1982 speech at Harvard University, "There is no such thing as a single-issue struggle because we don't live single-issue lives."

Dorothy Roberts's now-classic book *Killing the Black Body: Race, Reproduction, and Meaning of Liberty* traces the ways in which black women's procreative liberties have been systematically attacked, suppressed, and ignored in American law, even as legal protections have been enacted that only benefit the privileged (especially middle-class, married white women).[116] Despite their vulnerability at the mercy of a hostile society, black women have a long and rich tradition with birthing, breastfeeding, and raising their children. Black midwives in the South, for example, have an unbroken record (unbroken, yet intentionally weakened by state officials) in providing skilled, knowledgeable, and holistic care to pregnant, birthing, and postpartum mothers.[117] The disruptions to breastfeeding are not the result of inferior mothering. Anthropologist Acquanda Stanford points out that the way in which most headlines and research reports relay breastfeeding statistics elides this fact. Language like "breastfeeding rates for black U.S. women . . . lag overall"[118] is meant to convey the problem of disparity, but the "measuring stick" is always white women, as Stanford notes.

I cannot emphasize enough that *intersectionality* is not meant to be a fashionable synonym for *diversity*; it has to do with oppression more than identity. For example, Imani identifies as a woman and as a mother, much as I do. On the other hand, our experiences with breastfeeding differ in part because we are women from divergent social histories with unequal access to privilege. She told me that she generally did not feel like a very privileged person, but because of her advanced education and the resulting upward economic mobility, she had the opportunity to discover and explore options like natural birth and breastfeeding, which seem unavailable to the rest of the people in her community and in her family.

This experience, not incidentally, has led her to pursue training as a doula, a birth assistant, for the black community. She wants to do pro-bono work with teenage mothers because, as she says, "an African American, eighteen-year-old girl, who is pregnant by herself, doesn't want a thirty-year-old, married, tall, blonde, stay-at-home mom telling her how to birth." The various axes of relative privilege to which Imani refers—race, age, class, appearance, and marital status—all shape access to better birth experiences. Note that breastfeeding can be an extension of the birth experience rather than an entirely separate experience.

Philosophers of science, such as Karen Barad, explicitly connect the social to the physical as part of the intersectionality concept.[119] Breastfeeders' experiences differ depending on social status *and* on the embodiment of that status. Systems of oppression intervene into the physical experience with breastfeeding (think of milk supply, breast and nipple shape, and degree of pain and pleasure). These same systems belie mothers' interpretations of their babies' physical needs and capacities (think of latch quality, sucking ability, digestion, weight gain, and fussiness). Medical providers treat breastfeeders differently—and breastfeeders' trust in doctors varies—depending on factors like age, race, class, and education. If milk production is an issue, a nurse may be more likely to hand a young black woman a supplemental bottle of formula but will call in lactation assistance for a married, middle-class white woman.[120] These different practices in turn can either diminish milk production by cutting off demand or enhance it by encouraging more breastfeeding.

Patricia Hill Collins theorizes that any lasting change to the layered systems of oppression will have to come from the margins, from those shut out from and divested from the dominant culture.[121] In this book, I delve into how exceptional breastfeeders like Imani resist and reshape expectations.

Renowned midwife and revered hippie elder Ina May Gaskin writes in *Ina May's Guide to Breastfeeding* that she and her colleagues on the Farm, a former commune established in 1971 and the current center of home birth midwifery, have always striven to take the lead of the mother and baby in dispensing any breastfeeding advice.[122] She delightedly describes a scientific study that identified more than fifty cues that babies give mothers to indicate their readiness to nurse. Now Ina May, as she is colloquially known, has proof of what she knew all along from experience with breastfeeding mothers. Had she waited for science, a generation of new mothers would have lost out on her wisdom; not only that, but it is likely that the scientists would not have even explored these questions without learning of these cues from breastfeeders and "lay" experts like Ina May in the first place. Science has a tendency to ignore experience unless it has been fully operationalized and tested; until then, some scientists seem to think that people are simply passing along a bunch of dippy old wives' tales.

Experiential knowledge matters at least as much as accepted institutional knowledge. But how do we interpret other people's experiences without explaining them away using our institutional (academic, medical, or scientific) perspectives? *Ethnography*, literally translated, means "writing culture." I am writing secrets and revealing intimacies. "I'm still breastfeeding him," Liza replied quietly. After I asked her the obvious next question, the whispered confession—"He's seven"—hung in the air as she awaited my response. Did she expect dismay? Incredulity? She got what I always give: unblinking, poker-faced passivity. It often unnerves people in my daily life. It shuts them down sometimes. Whether it is because they think I am bored or unimpressed or whether they think I am silently judging them with the harshest criticisms they have always feared might be wielded against them, I do not know. It may not be a positive quality in an ethnographer. I have seen researchers who ask naive questions, unafraid of their own ignorance and nosiness, endear themselves to their interlocutors. Sometimes the real experts (the old, colonialist term is *study subjects*) want to reach out and patiently correct the uninitiated, teach them what's what, and set the record straight. When I am interviewing someone and find I have fallen into this unhelpful habit of mine, I might jump in with a confession of my own to even the score, to seem more accessible and to put them at ease (these efforts are intermittently successful). I want their trust more than anything. I know I will be reporting, contextualizing, and interpreting their secrets. My greatest fear is betraying secrets by conveying them in the wrong way, sharing someone else's secret, putting their vulnerable information out there and having others dismiss them as oddballs—or worse, having the readers of my research decide that somebody needs to put a stop to what these folks are doing. I can hear the medical, authoritarian protestations in my head: "How dare they breastfeed a child for so long? That is child abuse!" Or, "What if these milk-sharing arrangements spread disease?" I hope to honor my interviewees' trust by providing enough context to promote better understanding, not judgment.

Part of decolonizing breastfeeding is realizing that our social science research tools (surveys, ethnography, in-depth interviews) delimit what we know—producing one kind of knowledge—just as the research tools in medicine (blood tests, brain scans, heart monitors) produce a different kind of knowledge.[123]

If gender is a performance, so too is breastfeeding/nursing. Instead of thinking of breastfeeding as a natural, preexisting physiology that we can observe dispassionately (perhaps taking note of interesting variations in this culture or that), we can imagine that it is created through the act of doing it. Judith Butler suggests we avoid "producing the subject."[124] She argues that men and women enact those roles, which they learn through social norms. Sociologists call it "doing gender."[125] If we say that there are always already such things as men and women—we produce them as subjects—just existing in nature, then we eliminate the possibility of something different. Queer theory hinges on the philosophy of questioning the subject.

Queering breastfeeding requires us to maintain fluidity in our definitions, to not cave to the scientific pressure to operationalize (to produce measurable subjects). The mothers and others who breastfeed in unconventional ways actively queer the concept. Let's start with some low hanging fruit: butch lesbians breastfeeding. Breastfeeding is so heavily associated with feminine performativity that some of the women I interviewed told me that they had failed as mothers, failed their sex, and failed as women when their bodies did not produce enough milk. Butches breastfeeding subvert this limiting, pain-inducing narrative in multiple disparate ways: by not performing other feminine gender norms, by constructing and renaming breastfeeding as a utilitarian "food delivery system," by flaunting it in public in part to upset the closed-minded, and by hiding it from medical authorities and even from family members.

Exceptional breastfeeding may normalize queer breastfeeding and queer normal breastfeeding. Critics might say that queer-identified individuals' breastfeeding is a version of *mainstreaming,* or giving up the benefits of queerness by engaging in conformity.[126] As we will see in the coming chapters, queer breastfeeding experiences can easily be routine, prosaic, and mostly confirming of the breastfeeding status quo. And a breastfeeder need not be queer in terms of gender or sexual identity to interrupt the prevailing discourse. An adoptive mother who suckles her baby with the help of an SNS filled with formula or a touch-averse woman who exclusively pumps her milk may upend conventional understandings of breast milk and breastfeeding.

Lanie, the mother of six whose son "nurses" his sister, used her experience to help other women with their breastfeeding: "I worked with a mom who didn't have a breast. I said, 'just energetically imagine that you have a breast and you have the source. You have it in you as you are feeding the bottle.'"

Others' Milk, I hope, can incite our imagination, as Lanie suggested, producing a less bounded world of breastfeeding—one that does not yet exist but perhaps could be coming.

THE ARC OF *OTHERS' MILK*

In chapter 2, "Cleavages," I explore the dimensions of breastfeeding difficulties, from mild and major anxieties to a range of crises and family interference. These include betrayals by bodies failing to produce milk as expected, by grandmothers who want to feed babies bottles of formula, and by employers who cannot see fit to accommodate pumping needs—in violation of the law and fundamental ethics. I then consider why and how breastfeeders persevere through these challenges in chapter 3, "The Mother of Invention." Why, when we have the option of serviceable simulacra (good-enough formula in organic, vitamin-balanced, and allergy-free varieties and dozens upon dozens of baby bottle models with varying nipple shapes and sizes from which to choose), do breastfeeders keep going, sometimes necessitating extraordinary measures? It comes down to the relative benefits—not so much in a cost-benefit, rational economic sense but in a kaleidoscope of outcomes that include a number of self-actualizing processes that help the breastfeeder as well as the baby. In the absence of a more collective existence, individuals persist with breastfeeding by concocting practical solutions and idiosyncratic narratives. It often takes enormous willpower and access to unconventional resources to make exceptional breastfeeding happen.

A major impediment and sometimes help to exceptional breastfeeders—depending on their social standing and their particular needs—are the authorities that represent the institutions of motherhood (e.g., La Leche League), medicine, and capitalism (see chapter 4, "Milking the System"). Part of breastfeeding through disruptions and around social barriers involves dealing with these authorities face-to-face, and exceptional breastfeeders employ a number of strategies to preserve their autonomy. From willfully confronting those in power to harnessing consumer power to ignoring and even lying to authorities, exceptional breastfeeders contest the validity of institutional aims over their very personal ones. Some become formally recognized as experts themselves to gain back some power. This contested arena politicizes exceptional breastfeeders, who, if they do not already view their breastfeeding as defiant, begin to embrace its politics either overtly or more subtly after experiencing conflict. Other breastfeeders should not have to go through these trials because breastfeeding is hard enough as it is, they reason.

Breastfeeding is thought of and experienced as natural and feminine, the most intense bonding practice between a loving mother and her helpless baby. But exceptional breastfeeders' experiences contradict these essentialist ideas. Nongestational parents breastfeeding or being masculine and breastfeeding disrupt the normative framework. Their breastfeeding is not bonding-lite. Just because they are not experiencing it as "femininity" or biological destiny does not make their breastfeeding experiences any less powerful than anyone else's. In chapter 5, "Busting Binaries," I closely examine breastfeeders' identity-making and gendered embodiment of motherhood and otherhood. While some breastfeeders understand the experience as the ultimate expression of feminine biopower, others work to dissociate breastfeeding, breasts, and breast milk from gender norms. Neither perspective is simple in the context of exceptional breastfeeding. Exceptional breastfeeders confront the layered meanings of their breasts: Are they sexual? Aesthetic? Utilitarian? The answers to these charged questions come from their lived experiences. They negotiate bonding as it relates to gender. When the milk comes from others, in a bottle, or both, what does that mean for their motherly instincts? Some openly deliberate the intersections of gender and their own breastfeeding, finding comfort and confidence along the way.

In chapter 6, "Fluidity of the Family," I track how exceptional breastfeeding serves to "make kin" in novel ways. I draw on Donna Haraway's concept of "kinnovation." Whether on purpose or without really meaning to, exceptional breastfeeders pioneer and rediscover collective ways to breastfeed, which bind them to others outside of the orthodox mother-baby dyad. Along with a distribution of increasing intimacy and duration, these practices can create casual kin (as in some milk-sharing relationships), affective relations (such as surrogates who remain "like family" with the parents), oddkin[127] (invented relationships like "breastfeeding" siblings), and other-mothering[128] (especially co-nursing comothers). Politicized exceptional breastfeeders champion their family forms.

Gender, family, and politics come together as exceptional breastfeeders forge solidarity, the topic of chapter 7, "'Outpouring of Support.'" Despite a social context that isolates exceptional breastfeeders—who have to fight public sentiment, institutional authority, family pressures, and their own psyches—their need to engage in adaptive and creative versions of breastfeeding actually helps them find one another. Out of necessity and out of a desire to improve matters for everyone, they reach out beyond their familiar circles. The mechanisms that help forge this solidarity—which could form the basis for a grassroots social movement—include inspiration-seeking, networking, perspective-taking, and an engagement of the rules of reciprocity. The exceptional breastfeeders come from all backgrounds, and their unconventional varieties of breastfeeding are widely divergent. But together, they have some power. They form a collective voice calling for greater support and a more flexible understanding of motherhood and otherhood, of gender, and of family and kinship and social relationships. The story is not about breastfeeding, ultimately, but about the exceptions that might change the rules.

2 · CLEAVAGES
Negotiating Challenges

A screaming baby at the breast was not the Madonna-esque image I had in mind.

—Sabine

I can't even figure out how to feed my kid. So I'm automatically a failure right out of the gate.

—Marilyn

"I figured, I have boobs, I have a baby, put the baby to my boob and there we go!" remembered Mona, a married lesbian and mother of two. Because her wife had a relatively easy time with breastfeeding their first child, Mona had no inkling that breastfeeding could be complicated. But it often is. She went on to say, "I never thought that I had to worry about latch, that I had to worry about how wide his mouth was open, that I had to worry about whether he was sucking. I guess naiveté was my worst enemy.... I feel bad for other women who are not as determined as I am to breastfeed, that they see that they are not doing it right and they just accept the formula. Maybe I'm too driven to my own demise and the baby's weight loss, but I was almost desperate to breastfeed."

Like many Americans, Mona did not grow up seeing any breastfeeding. She lives in a rural, mostly Latinx area of California with limited access to the kinds of outsourced supports[1] like lactation consultants and support groups that thrive in middle-class suburbs and urban communities. The U.S. breastfeeding rate has climbed steadily upward over the past few years with 81.1 percent of babies "ever breastfed" (even once) in 2013 compared to 76.1 percent in 2009.[2] Studies credit baby-friendly hospital initiatives

(BFHIs), which generally include greater access to lactation consultants.[3] Still, plenty of motivated breastfeeders who encounter trouble are largely left to figure it out by themselves.

Mona, whose thyroid condition limited her milk production, preferred breast milk to formula for her baby; it was cheaper, more nutritious, and protective against stomach ailments and colds—and it was "her motherly duty to provide," she said. Several doctors advised formula, which left Mona "feeling devastated." She cried so much that she could not bring herself to travel to the La Leche League (LLL) meetings her cousin told her about. When a friend at work overheard Mona's concerns about the baby's weight, the coworker interjected, "Hey, I'm overproducing!" and offered her extra milk. Mona told me, "I had never heard of it. At first, I was just like, 'That is the weirdest thing ever,' but he was six pounds and twelve ounces. I knew he needed somebody else's milk."

Only 44.4 percent of U.S. breastfeeders still breastfeed exclusively by the time their infants reach three months of age.[4] Presumably, the rest either supplement with formula or only provide formula. But people like Mona, who supplemented with breast milk only, might self-report exclusively as "breastfeeding" if they understand giving breast milk to mean the same thing as breastfeeding. Others might check a box marked "mixed feeding" if they feed their baby another person's donated milk in a bottle. In any case, those high numbers of breastfeeders who attempt it cannot always keep going even if they want to. They have to contend with a number of barriers.[5] And their goals can be indistinct and flexible, especially if they are trying to create a breastfeeding relationship for the first time.

Westerners tend to fetishize individualism and personal rights, a preoccupation that extends back to the Enlightenment. The culture fosters pride in individuals striking out on their own and surviving all sorts of trials by themselves. But breastfeeding is a communal effort—from being taught how to initiate it (how to latch and how to hold a nursing baby) to having help getting meals and rest and taking care of other children in order to nurse frequently. Lisette helped her daughter breastfeed: "I didn't leave her side for four months. . . . It was intense, but we got through it. Most people would give up. You had to have somebody there to hold [the baby] so she could lie down. I said [to my daughter], 'Quit your job.'" Only a small percentage of women can afford to stay out of the paid labor market, and they still need help. Lactation consultants and doulas can be great, but they are neither free nor accessible to all. And hospitals usually discharge mothers soon after birth (which is not always a bad thing). There is no universal workable system of support.

To this weak support structure, one can add the formidable weight of anxiety in a context where mothers are supposed to be "natural" at the job. Others can compound the uncertainty by seeming to thwart and second-guess breastfeeders' every effort, and unforeseen emergencies and crises arise as additional stumbling blocks. Breastfeeders may find the relationship harmonious and pleasant when all goes swimmingly with the latch, the milk production, and the baby's growth, but even trouble-free breastfeeding can be difficult to reconcile with one's need for bodily independence and control.[6] Exceptional breastfeeders have to traverse some particularly rocky terrain among a confounding array of physical, social, structural, and personal limitations.

A SPECTRUM OF ANXIETIES

"I was more scared about breastfeeding than I was [about] giving birth," Peggy, a Canadian administrative assistant and breastfeeding mother of two, told me. And though she knew she would get a year of paid leave after the birth (a necessity not afforded to most U.S. parents), she still worried about how hard it would be and whether she was up to it. Breastfeeders, lacking an adequate blueprint, can be quite apprehensive. They ask themselves: Will I be able to do it? Will my milk be enough? Can I last six months or a year? What will my baby's needs be? What will others think?

Tales of woe are common, made worse by the high stakes.[7] An ethnographic study of middle-class breastfeeding mothers found that breastfeeding signifies, for them, a commitment to the mother-child relationship.[8] It may also serve as outward evidence of self-determined mothering, proof that they are "independent freethinkers" who do not go down the well-trod path of the formula-filled bottle.[9] One now-veteran breastfeeder I interviewed, Kiki, thought breastfeeding was a "nightmare" at first; the suffering led her to *hate* motherhood itself. If she could not breastfeed, then why even bother with any of it? She could not perceive the initial trouble as a routine, correctable complication at first. Instead, her inability to endure the "agonizing" pain meant she was a failure, not a committed mother.

Lactation experts call getting started with breastfeeding "initiation," and the other meaning of the word is appropriate too. Those first few days and weeks can feel like "hell week" in some fraternity's hazing ritual. Ellen expected breastfeeding to go well. Her plans went awry: "[The nurses] just kept taking him away, so we never really learned breastfeeding. They tried to get him to latch; we tried to breastfeed for, like, two weeks with a nipple shield and just breast-exclusive. But then I quit trying because he wasn't latching on. I was getting really sick. I was using the nipple shield improperly. I had a 104° fever; it was crazy.... Postpartum, we were just spiraling out of control."

Ellen, beside herself with feelings of failure and a breast infection, gave up. Baby Ollie received bottles of formula from then on. Then one day, the baby just happened to latch on to her arm and she felt him sucking. She remembered, "I just was immediately like 'whoa,' so I put him to the breast. He started sucking. He nursed for the first time." Grateful and now enamored of breastfeeding, Ellen went on to nurse her son for two and a half years. She also donated her extra milk to those who were not so lucky. In its broad strokes, this sequence of events is typical of exceptional breastfeeders: difficulty, solution, and then helping others along.

MILK SURVEILLANCE AND NARRATIVES OF ENOUGH

Among the many vexing aspects of breastfeeding, milk quality and quantity and flow speed have unique powers to preoccupy everyone involved (except perhaps the child). Breastfeeders cannot predict or even fully control how their lactation will go. They may mitigate this loss of control by carefully monitoring and measuring their milk, becoming somewhat dispassionate observers, like scientists studying their own bodies. There is a contradiction here: they also have to be loving providers. At times, they may feel more like milk producers than mothers and parents.[10] Sociologist Linda Blum points out that all this focus on milk, removed from the mother, alienates breastfeeders and serves the patriarchal interest in controlling women's bodies.[11] These self-studying breastfeeders collect evidence of their milk quantity and quality to prove that they are good enough providers and thus good enough parents.

Breast milk itself has become a value-added commodity—literally in some contexts (when exchanged for money) but mostly metaphorically: it is "liquid gold," priceless and precious, so good for humanity that people must give every drop to their baby or else generously offer it to others for free.[12] A new milk-collecting cup on the market allows breastfeeders to collect any excess milk spilling from the one breast while the infant suckles the other side. A mother posting online enthused, "No more wasting milk on the nursing pad!" Some breastfeeding scholars recommend getting rid of the "gold standard" idea.[13] It makes breastfeeding sound out of reach and aspirational, appropriate only in just the right circumstances rather than a regular, accessible part of childrearing for everyone. As it stands, when breastfeeders encounter trouble with breastfeeding, many feel it as an insult to their worth.

Breast pump design improvements from the 1990s to the present have made it ever easier to keep track of output.[14] Efficient pumps with attached bottles that double as graduated cylinders bring forth milk that had heretofore been difficult to measure. In language borrowed from economics—supply, demand, shortage, stockpile, distribution, efficiency, flow, surplus, quality control—society positions breast-pumping caregivers as both labor and management. The desire to establish a stockpile in the freezer as insurance against any supply shortages in the future leads to the purchase of extra freezers in the garage and the borrowing of friends', neighbors', and family members' freezer space. These freezer stashes provide tangible proof of success and require competent and careful handling. Based on my observations of breastfeeders' relationships with their milk, it seems that there is an ongoing moral panic over whether one's milk is "enough." Some cope better than others and model ways to become satisfied that one's milk and, by extension, one's mothering is enough.

Supply Curve

Latisha, a medical technician and divorced mother of two, was the first in her family to breastfeed. "I stopped breastfeeding around four months because, in my mind, I thought I wasn't getting enough milk when I was. There was just a lack of knowledge and the lack of support," she remembered. She constantly needed to stop her family members from giving cereal supplements to her second child, whom she ended up breastfeeding for a year. She explained that her family members are black southerners who "believe in feeding the child." With breastfeeding, nobody knows exactly how much milk the baby gets. But with cereals, formula, or pumped milk, the quantity is comfortingly clear. The cereals reduced her child's suckling, which, in turn, signaled Latisha's body to produce less milk. She eventually figured out a way to reassure her elders: she would squeeze her secondborn's chunky little legs as proof that he was well fed.

Sometimes even being able to see evidence of plenty is not enough. There is no shortage of eye-popping pics online of rows upon rows of Medela- or Lansinoh-brand storage bags full of "liquid gold" on display in their chilly vaults. There is also a veritable internet competition to see how many gallons of pumped milk donors can provide. Eve decided to donate her milk when her baby died soon after birth; she said it helped her grieve to be able to provide for other babies. Though proud that she donated twenty gallons, Eve admitted that her contribution paled in comparison to the hundreds of gallons from other donors she saw reported online. Even though individual breastfeeders may produce "too much"—or more than they need, anyway—there remains a cultural sense that there is never enough milk.

Different histories of breastfeeding contribute to this sensibility of scarcity. Aster, a Latina mother of two living in California, attributed her mother's and her aunts' supplement-pushing to their memories of being unable to provide sufficient breast milk—or even enough food—to their children back in Mexico due to extreme poverty. This intergenerational food insecurity feeds into the mind-set that "the more you feed the baby, the better," as Emie, a Latina lactation consultant, phrased it.

Trying to fill breast pump bottles to the highest possible number of ounces can be nerve-wracking. (And lactation consultants will warn that being nervous can reduce the body's ability to release milk.) I induced lactation sans pregnancy or advanced preparation when my second adoptive son arrived without warning (nobody knew his birth mother was pregnant). An inveterate minimalist, I had just given away every last baby item in my house. While a friend rushed over to install a sham crib that we would need to satisfy the social worker's home inspection (I planned on cosleeping against the rules), I waited around for a lactation consultant at the hospital to help me learn how to establish a milk supply. I pumped my breasts for half an hour every two hours with a noisy hospital-grade pump plugged into an outlet at home. Because I also needed to breastfeed my baby frequently, I installed myself in an oversized chair that accommodated me, my new baby, my thirteen-month-old and his toys, and all the hoses, flanges, tape, cream, and tubes I would need for pumping and supplementing with a supplemental nursing system (SNS). I did not always bother to put on a shirt, as many a houseguest would discover. My friend Wendy Simonds photographed me in my new habitat: "Say 'moo!'" she told me.

To nudge my milk production, I took the drug domperidone and the herb fenugreek, which had the odd side effect of making my perspiration smell like maple syrup. Little Leo nursed constantly, or so it seemed. The bottles began to have a bit more in them each time I pumped, and after a few months, my son began to be satisfied at the breast without the need for supplementation.

But a new quantity problem cropped up when I went back to work after an unpaid six months at home. I found myself needing to pump between teaching my classes in order to keep my body producing any milk. I literally ran to my office, (politely?) pushing past students-with-just-one-quick-question to pump both sides simultaneously during the passing time. I also used this time to eat, restoring the necessary calories. While I did not keep a log, like some of the more fastidious breastfeeders I interviewed, I did report my output to my family and friends each day, always aiming to best my rather paltry record of four ounces. I did a little dance one day when I managed to squeeze out that much from the always better producing left side.

The capitalism-rooted compulsions to self-monitor and to achieve, to compete, and to value production contribute to breastfeeders' feelings of inadequacy as parents. There is never enough milk—even when there is an oversupply—because there are competitions to pump the most, to display the most, to give away the most. We get into even more trouble when output becomes proof of maternal legitimacy. Insufficient milk means not measuring up to feminine expectations. It can feel like being out of touch with one's body—and worse, out of sync with one's baby, putting "good" motherhood status in peril. Some exceptional breastfeeders, though, work these binds loose for everyone.

Enough Is as Good as a Feast

Sometimes low supply is a deeply unpleasant surprise, but in my case and for Mira, a mother of four, it is to be expected. Mira knew she would have to deal with low milk supply even though her ill-informed doctors attempted to allay her fears: "I have insufficient glandular tissue. My mom does too. My

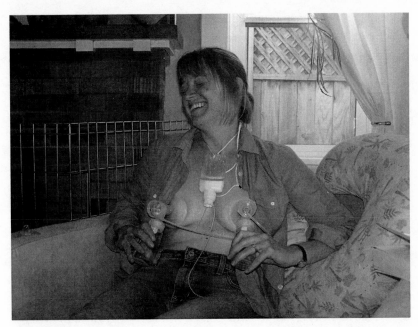

Say "Moo!"

aunt also. Growing up, I knew my mom did not make enough. That my aunt didn't make enough. That it was very obvious once I hit puberty, mine were lopsided. My left side never really developed. My right side had some form but not a whole lot of definition. . . . I had asked the doctors about it, [and] they had said, 'Every woman can. Don't worry about it. Size doesn't matter.'"

Mira embarked on breastfeeding prepared. She knew her family history better than her doctors did, and she already had fraught, embodied experience with her underdeveloped breasts. She managed with some tools from capitalism: the right equipment and a can-do attitude. She routinely fed her baby before she even finished her shopping at Target: "The Lact-Aid [SNS] became my third boob, and I got so good at whipping that thing out, and nobody ever noticed!" In contrast to the never-enough discourse, for her, even *some* breast milk is enough—the baby gets the connection, the baby gets her immunities, and the baby gets some of the ideal nutrition. With the formula that Mira mixed with her own pumped milk, the baby received enough food. Mira contended with the prevailing assumption that formula is inadequate nutrition by inoculating it with her own powerful milk. She headed off any worries about bonding by keeping the baby to breast and integrating this adaptive form of breastfeeding into her workaday public life. A few more confident SNS users in enough Target stores, and this exceptional breastfeeding style could tip toward "normal."

Sanity Checks

Amy, on the other hand, got blindsided by low supply. Ironically, her mother has been a lifelong La Leche leader, and even she could not help. Amy consulted with five lactation experts and multiple doctors, hydrated all day long, took herbal remedies, ingested galactagogues (food and supplements thought to increase milk production), and used prescription medications, including domperidone and the nastier Reglan—a drug that tends to wreak havoc on one's hormones.[15] She dedicated months to trying to decipher this bodily mystery, all to no avail: "My plan was all along to breastfeed. It ended up that no matter how much I nursed and pumped around the clock, I never felt my milk increase. I never felt I had a supply. I didn't even know when my milk came in. It was kind of a mystery. I never felt any growth. I never got engorged. I looked. I couldn't see anything dripping out." She experienced "all this demand but no supply," telling me, "There are recommendations of how much the baby needs to gain, so I was weighing him." She began checking his weight after each feeding. After many weeks of an intensive pumping regimen, she realized that the numbers were not improving. She was upset by this stasis but happy to ditch the ineffectual pump. Her stress levels improved. But even after reluctantly turning to formula supplementation, she weighed her son at least weekly for what she called "sanity checks." Managing the numbers helped her get a handle on matters.

Amy collected evidence that she used to convince herself and others that her low supply was "real"; so much advice on breastfeeding rejects this possibility. Clinical researchers maintain that insufficient milk production is not the problem breastfeeders imagine it to be. These experts recommend a "self-efficacy" scale to measure "maternal confidence" and other "psychosocial" factors that account for whether the parent of a newborn continues or gives up on breastfeeding.[16] They suggest that breastfeeders with high self-efficacy—the ability to manage their bodies and feel confident about it—have fewer breastfeeding problems. These researchers call on service providers to do more to buoy breastfeeders' confidence. But this self-efficacy perspective can be read in another way: the success or failure of breastfeeding is up to the individual. Sometimes individuals feel like their service providers do not believe them when they report their breastfeeding problems. Amy and others with low supply complained to me about dogma proclaimed by experts and La Leche, which insists that everyone who gives birth can make enough milk. While it is certainly true that *most* breastfeeders are capable of making enough milk to exclusively breastfeed for up to a year, Amy truly could not.

Breastfeeders receive mixed messages from their medical providers, who until recently commonly referred to growth charts based on populations of formula-fed babies. Generally speaking, breastfed infants do not gain weight along the same trajectory as formula-fed babies.[17] Pediatricians might scare inexperienced breastfeeders into thinking that their milk production is lacking and thus to blame for their babies being behind the curve—when, in fact, the babies' weights are perfectly healthy. Any kind of stress, including anxiety about milk supply, can inhibit production.[18] Formula supplementation can diminish breast milk supply, further compounding a breastfeeder's perception that her body cannot produce enough milk. Other clinical research shows that breastfeeders experience "pressure" and "guilt" when their medical providers advise exclusive breastfeeding as the best way to fix their perceived supply problems.[19] Someone like Amy, who kept hearing that she just was not trying hard enough—that her self-efficacy and maternal confidence were the primary problems—felt terrible when her body refused to produce sufficiently despite her most determined efforts. Such caregivers may respond with all sorts of "sanity checks," careful monitoring of their efforts to prove to themselves that are not imagining their milk production problems.

Thad, a fifty-one-year-old transman who breastfed his two children years ago (he does not use the newer term *chestfeeding*), noted with relief that his second child put on weight more readily than the first: "Not having to deal with people going, 'Oh, he's losing weight; we've got to *worry* about him if he doesn't gain weight!' It's kind of like ay-yi-yi. Because they were threatening, well, 'We might have to put him on formula.'" As a parent who was both dedicated to breastfeeding and who had previous experience with unwanted formula-pushing, Thad had dealt with enough second-guessing.

Breastfeeders and medical personnel alike have been duped, breastfeeding advocates contend, by the normalization of formula and baby cereals. Historian Jill Lepore points out the suspicious coincidence of women suddenly running out of their own breast milk once artificial milk became available in the U.S. market.[20] The promotion of formula by its manufacturers, and by medical institutions shilling for them, contributed to a panic. Anthropologists and clinical researchers question the phenomenon of insufficient milk, arguing that it is rare to be unable to produce enough milk.[21] Anthropologists characterize it as something of a culture-bound syndrome, a symptom of urban life under capitalism, which is not conducive to the kind of frequent feeding humans have evolved to do. Whether low supply (still one of the most common reasons for quitting breastfeeding) is real or imagined—or a combination of the two—continues to be a matter of debate.[22] The question of low supply is like asking whether being gay is intrinsic and provable by science. It may be unanswerable, and it does not matter to the experience. It is also like demonstrations of concern for "obese" people. You have to wonder how much of the concern is about health and how much is a moralizing (and demoralizing) attack. Partly because of this controversy about milk production, breastfeeders with supply challenges need frequent reassurance that they can trust their bodies.

For Amy, the subtext of the dictum "anyone can breastfeed" implied that she was not trying hard enough despite the quantifiable evidence to the contrary. Giving formula, as she did, has its own learning curve: the right bottle position, the best shape and flow speed of the nipple, cost management, keeping it in stock, dealing with the baby's gas and constipation, finding the ideal product that the baby will tolerate, remembering to carry the necessary items everywhere, and so on.

Close measurement and monitoring of milk can weaken breastfeeders' confidence *or* bolster it. Exclusive pumpers deal with many of same challenges as other breastfeeders and maintain rigorous pumping schedules on top of everything else. Susan, a mother of three, stopped to pump before she went anywhere, and it took time: "I am pumping for about three hours, and I'm usually bagging milk and washing bottles for, like, forty-five minutes per day." Keeping track helped Susan prove that she was a dedicated mother. She said, "I like to measure it all out. I am kind of a numbers freak. I have everything I've pumped put into an app on my phone. And every time I've pumped, I keep running a timer. I am going to have all these numbers of how much I pumped, how many times I pumped, and all this other stuff." Amy and Susan had to remind themselves, and everyone else, that they were not taking the easy way out by using bottles; their output proved it. These mothers felt like their "sanity" was in question when their breastfeeding did not follow expectations. Through their sanity checks, they amassed proof that they were indeed good mothers.

Excess or Abundance?

Those whose bodies make more than enough milk face their own sets of problems and body management protocols. Milk letdowns sometimes produce a pins-and-needles feeling, engorgement is painful, and full breasts leak. Worse is the susceptibility to infections like mastitis, which Sherry, a birth doula and overproducer, described as being "hit by a train."

When a breastfeeder's body does not cooperate, it can make a person feel alienated from herself and from the baby. Ellen told me, "I just have so much milk. No matter how much I use compression and try to tell my body to slow down, my body was just making milk for six babies." Her infant daughter choked and gagged on the "fast, crazy-strong flow" of milk (called "overactive letdown"). Ellen tried chest compression and block nursing, wherein she offered either the left or the right breast at a given feeding session and only for a limited "block" of time. She needed to pump to relieve painful engorgement, but doing so increased the supply. Pumps suck. They can be powerful at extracting milk—and, for many, they are a pain to use. Some overproducers stick to hand expression to minimize the signal to the body to keep making more.

Ellen had such a strong flow that her baby could not stay latched onto the breast. Babies need the comfort of sucking, and this is where pacifiers (and fingers) come in. Some experts tell breastfeeders, without a shred of irony, that they should not cave in to their babies' demands and nurse too often, lest their (conniving?) babies "use them" as a pacifier. This topsy-turvy reasoning fails to recognize that it is the pacifier being used as a substitute breast, not the other way around. This attitude is an example of the social "boundaries of touch,"[23] which enforce limits on physical contact and treat parent-child intimacy with suspicion. Breastfeeders can be of two minds about it. A pacifier, while separating a baby from a warm breast temporarily, can avoid the spluttering and spitting up that come with a fire-hose milk flow. Pacifiers soothe without the risk of overfeeding the baby, and their use helps prevent cracked, bleeding nipples.

Breast milk does not have to become a Goldilocks conundrum where the flow or the supply is too much or too little. For some, these variations are manageable obstacles that come with the territory. Allie, who cofed her baby in partnership with her lesbian wife, laughed off the protocol of block feeding: "Someone was like, 'Oh, you know, you drain one side, and then you switch to the other.' And I'm like, 'I've never depleted one side. I've never not had milk.' My lactation consultant said, 'You could have fed Africa.' I was overly abundant. I pump-pump-pump because it was just like, 'Oh my god! Oh my god!' A huge supply."

Allie, and some other exceptional breastfeeders I interviewed, experienced the body's mystique, its very unpredictability, as part of the fun. Whereas low supply feels mostly like an affliction, oversupply can mean different things. When blamed for babies' reflux and choking, breastfeeders and experts may characterize it as pathological. "Abundance" puts a positive spin on a big milk supply. For Allie, the "huge supply" made it seem like there was always enough for everyone, including her baby and families in need of her milk donations.

Nutritional Value

Breastfeeders dutifully monitor their milk *quality*, tapping into narratives of not just "enough" but "good enough." Breast milk is subject to the widespread (though distinctly middle-class) ideology of *nutritionism*— the reduction of foods' value to their vitamin content and calorie count.[24] Every food we ingest, in this way of thinking, should have nutritional value. By eating these foods, our bodies themselves have more value, we are more morally upright, and we are good citizens taking charge and managing our health. Healthy eaters can contrast themselves with the exploited characters on poor-shaming reality television shows like *Here Comes Honey Boo-Boo*, where the plus-sized matriarch, Mama June, is the butt of the joke. My friends at the gym allow themselves to be temporarily "bad" once per week on their "cheat day" when they can eat foods of poor nutritional and moral substance. This pervasive view on morally correct diets influences breastfeeding.

But breast milk is rarely just a food. Besides having high-grade nutritional value, it is also thought to be "liquid love," suffused with medicinal and therapeutic qualities. Formula, in this framing, is processed food like potato chips. Ariel, a California-based homemaker and mother of one, explained, "I just don't like the idea of giving her something that is unnatural. The ingredients in the formula these days—I just don't like it. It is so disgusting.

If you ever smell it, it smells horrible." Other breastfeeders I talked with called formula "gross," "unethical," "unhealthy," and "risky." "People don't realize the risks of formula feeding on a population scale. The fact that it's a massive experiment in babies' health. It's never been actually trialed," said Lonny, a midwife and tandem-nursing mother from the United Kingdom. Even though formulas often sport labels that attest to the medicine-like benefits—such as the presence of fatty acids or oligosaccharides—the U.S. Food and Drug Administration (FDA) indeed does not test formula.

There are only a few randomized clinical studies on feeding babies formula versus breast milk. But there is some observational research on how formula-fed children fare health-wise compared to those who were breastfed or given breast milk.[25] Early benefits of breastfeeding include fewer ear infections and digestive problems in infancy; long-term benefits may include lower blood pressure and lower risk of diabetes, obesity, asthma, and eczema, as well as "cognitive benefits" like higher IQ.[26] The results are far from consistent, and the studies are often small or insufficient in their design. The science comes under fire from all sides. Some feminist observers argue that the probreastfeeding scientists bias the results and oversell the benefits of breastfeeding, and other feminists fault scientists for being biased in not bothering to investigate breastfeeding thoroughly enough.[27] Both worry that mothers and other caregivers do not get solid information with which to make their feeding decisions.

It can be quite difficult to show that breastfeeding is what makes the difference in babies' health when many other factors are at play. Further, is it just the breast milk or the holistic practice of breastfeeding that brings the benefits? Biological anthropologist Katie Hinde emphasizes that the act of suckling breast milk triggers two-way hormonal signals that serve as catalysts for changing the molecular and nutritional content of the milk.[28] This sort of scientific knowledge of breastfeeding can help feminists convince policy makers to eliminate the barriers to breastfeeding and to institute *real* help like paid leave from work (as opposed to more limited, employer-friendly—but still helpful—measures like free breast pumps and dedicated pumping space at work). Scientific proof that breastfeeding does wonders for some does not have to mean that alternatives to normative breastfeeding are inferior, or that pumping milk for a baby makes a person less devoted to mothering.

Food Safety

Many milk donors attest to their clean living habits in online posts offering surplus milk. In the interest of "full disclosure," they often note any
medications or alcohol consumption. Some may even report seemingly
less significant details like minor lapses in their veganism that are unlikely
to make much difference in the milk's composition. Posts on the website
onlythebreast.com, a rare venue for selling—rather than donating—breast
milk, sometimes include dubious "test results" that verify the milk's caloric
content and/or the lactating individual's genetic superiority. Breastfeeders
may offer "enhanced" milk for sale. Because breast milk is supposedly an
elixir that can improve athletic performance,[29] the ads may include DNA
analyses that reveal desirable ratios of fast twitch to slow twitch muscle
fibers,[30] among other qualities.

Milk banks, which are more conventional distributors—the ones in the
United States, Canada, and Mexico are certified by professionals running
the Human Milk Banking Association of North America (HMBANA)—
reject milk suspected of being dangerous or inadequate. They maintain
quality control by requiring blood tests (to rule out HIV and other com-
municable diseases)[31] and by screening donors for lifestyle factors that
could potentially contaminate the milk. Following agreed-upon protocols,
HMBANA milk banks exclude donations from the sick, smokers, heavy
drinkers, and those on certain medications. They discover these disqualify-
ing factors through self-reports on a questionnaire. Rhonda, a single mother
living in New York City, had her milk rejected by several milk banks because
she had lived in Germany for three years as a child when her father was sta-
tioned there with the Army. There is a small possibility that she could have
been exposed to mad cow disease, the pathogens for which can lie dormant
in the body, only to be transmitted in breast milk years later. The likelihood
of disease transmission is not enough to warrant any public health warn-
ings against breastfeeding one's own offspring, however. The milk is good
enough for her children but not for others, a rejection she called "annoying."

Milk bank staff members pasteurize and microbe-test accepted milk.
Once checked, sterilized, and packaged as "safe," they distribute it based on
a hierarchy of need: first to neonatal intensive care units (NICUs) and then
to those with a prescription. Apparently, these institutions grapple with
how much weight to give factors of "individual choice" against what they

determine to be "community benefit."[32] A request for milk for infants with no problematic medical conditions is a matter of individual choice. Those babies' lives are not at risk if they have formula. But potentially saving the lives of premature infants with "donor milk therapy" is considered a community benefit.[33]

Peer-to-peer milk donors and recipients may institute their own safeguards. They sterilize by flash pasteurizing[34] at home, conduct informal interviews or engage in amateur detective work (like checking out a donor's Facebook profile), deal only with friends of friends or others in their professional network, and—my personal favorite—discover a hobby or personal detail that vouches for the other person by virtue of apparent similarity to themselves. (She knits too? Well then, her milk is sure to be safe!) To be clear, recipients not only concern themselves with risk but also want to know if the other mother or caregiver is "healthy," a vague and subjective (and moral) standard.

Quality Standards

Breastfeeders worry about getting their babies the appropriate ratio of watery, thirst-quenching foremilk and dense, nutrient-rich hindmilk. At the breastfeeding support groups I observed, there was much confusion about how to ascertain the difference and how to time and pace feedings to ensure that the baby receives the ideal "dosage" of each type of milk. On different occasions, several breastfeeders noted that their pumped milk seemed too watery. Was the baby better than the pump at getting the good hindmilk, and was that why they could not see the proof of it? They have to rely on whatever clues they can get—however slapdash—in order to effectively monitor the quality. Is the baby gaining enough weight? Does the baby's hunger seem satisfied this time? Do my breasts feel drained right now? It's enough to drive breastfeeders to distraction when they lack tangible, definitive evidence that their bodies are up to snuff.

Cricket had high amounts of the digestive enzyme lipase in her milk, which caused it to change soon after pumping or taken from the freezer. It is a common condition that lactation consultants diagnose easily; that's how Cricket learned of its name. She said, "I had to smell to see which ones are good and which ones had gone bad. I have since read, and I probably had read it then, just because it smells rancid doesn't mean that she [her daughter] still wouldn't have taken it. But I have a certain quality-control threshold. I wasn't willing to serve my daughter rancid milk." Trusting herself over authoritative advice that says that high lipase milk is not "rancid," Cricket would rather throw it out than give her child anything less than the freshest, best quality. Exercising her discriminating taste also improved her feelings of maternal success. She could put her judicious decision-making skills to work. She regained a sense of control in the face of her body's transgression.

Risk Management

"I have a life to protect," said Tayshia. This statement explains why she was meticulous about her diet while breastfeeding, which she continued until her daughter turned four. Experts unwittingly encourage this obsession by asking breastfeeders to consider their milk content as the potential cause of their infants' indigestion. Breastfeeders endure elimination diets, swear off foods they love, and reluctantly eat foods they dislike all in a sometimes tail-chasing effort to improve their milk quality and prevent their babies' intestinal gas, spitting up, diarrhea, apparent discomfort, constipation, and/or excessive crying. The infant son of a pair of cofeeding lesbian mothers from New York, Kelly and Marybeth, suffered gastrointestinal problems from food allergies and had eczema: "We both went on a total elimination diet while we were breastfeeding for approximately an eternity. But I think it was a year. More than a year? [turning to her partner] She thinks it was more than a year. Somewhere between a year and an eternity where we basically ate like three things for a very long time, and we introduced things one at a time until we were sure that he wasn't reacting to them."

Instead of reaching for formula, these two mothers turned to the scientific method, conducting control-variable experiments on themselves and their baby. They thought of milk as an essentially mild and natural food, which is why they did not try any varieties of hypoallergenic formula. Their baby was just especially sensitive, requiring greater care and attention that they were willing and able to provide. Intentional diets are a worthwhile burden to some breastfeeders. Kelly and Marybeth went to these lengths in response to their baby's allergy symptoms, but other breastfeeders do so for less immediate reasons. For example, Tayshia, a vegan, pursued the cleanest diet possible and ate spicy foods in part to introduce them to her baby via breast milk. She pointed out that as a breastfeeder, she cannot "manage the formula factory," but she can manage her own body.

Bailey sought donor milk for her deceased sister's infant twins who were undernourished at the time of their mother's death. Neither twin could stomach formula, but one child was especially sensitive, and so Bailey headed to the internet for help. She looked for "mass donors," she said, because she and her husband "wanted the babies to get used to certain diets." The wildly different diets of "one hundred" donors could have perpetuated the infants' digestive problems. Bailey's motives included the infants' survival, of course, but she also wanted to honor her sister's beliefs about breast milk being best. Convenience was also a factor: it is certainly easier to manage a few large donations than many smaller ones. But the meager science on the impact of breastfeeders' diets on babies' health does not uphold Bailey's assumption that bland, unchanging diets equal easier-to-digest milk nor does it support Tayshia's assumption that a spicy diet makes the breastfed child into an adventurous eater later on.[35] (One study did find a general association between breastfeeding and a decline in picky eating in toddlers, however.[36]) Controlling diets and thus controlling milk goes way beyond the well-known rules about limiting alcohol, caffeine, and drugs to include staying away from ice cream and strawberries, for example. These dedicated caregivers apply diverse commonsense understandings about diets and digestion to breastfeeding. It is part of the total motherhood project to reduce any and all risks.

Prescription in hand, and using funds I had been saving for an adoption, I purchased thousands of three-ounce bottles of milk bank milk for Evan, my elder son, over the course of his first year. Every week or so, I drove the thirty miles to the milk bank to pick up a batch. I waited in the front of the portable building as the employees packed the cute, squat, glass bottles in a cooler. I was once introduced to the bank's white-coated "chemist," who I usually spotted busily filling bottles or pasteurizing trays of them. Occasionally, another mother would be there reading a magazine, hooked up to one of the pumps provided in an office cubby, patiently offering her milk.

Some batches were redolent with pinto beans; others gave off a mildly floral aroma (I have no idea why); some had a more neutral milky scent. To my mind, with each new cap I unscrewed, fitted with a nipple, and placed in his mouth, he was getting a multivitamin and an introduction to flavors and untold immunity boosters. It surprises me now to think that I did not wonder even once if any of the milk contained traces of medication or toxins or pathogens. Like many milk recipients, I reflexively trusted the donors and the milk bank. And when I received milk from friends, I just assumed optimal quality. I spent the money on the milk not because I thought formula was bad but because I had some savings. I reasoned that my baby had a rough start—his birth mother had been homeless and addicted to drugs and alcohol while she was pregnant with him—so why not bet on the possibility that the milk would live up to at least some of the hype?

Purity and Contamination

Some people worry about breast milk purity—maybe too much. A small research study conducted by a public health scholar and published in the medical journal *Pediatrics* in 2013[37] created an uproar: media outlets that caught wind of the study promptly penned scary headlines like *USA Today*'s "Buying Milk Online? It Might Be Contaminated."[38] Scholars who studied online breast milk sharing were more circumspect. There were problems with the ethics and the methodology of the *Pediatrics* study, starting with the researchers' lying to the sellers about the milk's purpose. The women selling the milk thought they were sending it to other mothers, not to a lab. The researchers also biased their interpretations by reporting the bacterial load of the shipped milk without comparing it to the bacteria on home-mixed bottles of formula—known to be more germ-ridden than pumped breast milk. The report neglected to mention that most informal milk sharing happens between people who know one another; most deliveries occur in person rather than by shipment; and hardly anyone sells the milk to strangers.[39] The fear-mongering conclusions from the study are highly questionable.

Still, a perspective of breast milk as dangerous and dirty persists. Naheema, a mother of three, said, "It's a body fluid. It's like sharing body fluids. [In a disgusted voice] I am a hypochondriac. I would not trust another woman's breast milk. I know this sounds crazy. That breast milk is for *your* baby. You know what I mean? It seems a little bit intimate sharing another person's body fluid, and I don't know if I would be comfortable allowing my child to. I don't even like hugging my husband when he is sweating [Laughs]." Naheema backtracked a little as she considered that she would, in fact, share breastfeeding with her sister if the need arose. Their familial and emotional closeness makes sharing body fluids more acceptable. She blamed her own neurosis for her rejection of milk sharing and insinuated that milk sharing is unnatural.

Which narrative will prevail? Will it be the one that says milk is a body fluid and potential vector for disease, a transmitter of illicit drugs, and a violation of personal boundaries—or just "gross," like sweat? Or will the story be that milk is pure, wholesome, and magical? Could the shift toward personalized medicine—genetics-based and microbiome-related treatment specific to individuals—work its way more thoroughly into the meanings we give to breast milk (i.e., "Breast milk is for *your* baby.")?

Ethnographic research suggests that breastfeeders tend to be careful with their milk.[40] Some caregivers label their milk to keep track of dietary changes and the perceived effects on the infant. Susan told me that she differentiated the baby's milk from her postcelebratory "margarita milk," which she designated "for pink-eye treatment only" (the inflammatory *Pediatrics* article notwithstanding, breast milk has well-documented antibacterial properties). She effectively separated the pure from the tainted. The lactation consultants I observed advised breastfeeding support group attendees to label and sort their freezer bags of milk by pump dates in order to always use the oldest first. When one of the consultants pointed out that quality diminishes over time, I immediately wondered whether some months-old freezer stashes would still be considered liquid gold. Maybe those bags should be called "liquid bronze" instead.

Scientific understandings about contaminants and contagions in breast milk are cloudy, as we have seen. Experts encourage breastfeeders who are sick with a cold or flu to nurse their babies in part because the milk contains virus-fighting agents that transfer to the nursling.[41] Interestingly, the saliva of sick babies seems to transmit signals to the body of anyone breastfeeding that child (whether or not that person is the gestational parent) to produce antibodies.[42] Sometimes milk fights germs, and sometimes it transfers them. HIV and some other infections like hepatitis sometimes pass into breast milk. Medicines and drugs that the breastfeeder takes may pose a problem, but the research on particular drugs can be lacking. It is no surprise that breastfeeders feel troubled. They do not want to do the wrong thing, but they never can be sure what is right.[43]

"Reasonable" amounts of the commonly used legal drugs caffeine and alcohol are not subject to pump-and-dump recommendations. But over and over again, I listened to breastfeeders in support groups anxiously ask about how much alcohol or caffeine or sugar or Tylenol they could safely consume and how long it took to reach the breast milk and so on. Lily, one of the breastfeeders I interviewed, expressed both pride and disappointment in her sister, who stopped using marijuana during pregnancy but chose not to breastfeed so that she could return to smoking. A roundup of the medical literature on marijuana's effects on breastfed babies found that the concern was on par with that of cigarette smoking and that there may be a slight slowdown in motor development.[44] Could it have been better overall for Lily's niece or nephew to receive nutritious breast milk and the closeness with the mother even if trace amounts of THC were passed along? For political (and misogynistic) reasons, there are minimal scientific studies of marijuana and too few studies of breast milk[45] to make an adequate guess. Uncertainty like this makes it so that some breastfeeders experience their lactating bodies as a source of life as well as a source of danger.

The mainstream view that cow's milk is wholesome, thanks to decades of marketing campaigns and government-approved food pyramids,[46] informs the general understanding of breast milk. Cow's milk consumption continues to be normative in the United States despite the prevalence of lactose intolerance or "maldigestion" (afflicting about 65 percent of the postinfancy population).[47] The ubiquity of breakfast cereal and the fact that milk is always on offer in elementary school lunches attest to its prevalence. Several counterdiscourses question milk's purity, however. Vegan activists and many others point to the unsanitary conditions of some dairy farms or the factory-like extraction from poorly treated, antibiotic- and hormone-contaminated cows. The more radical critics cast the substance as unfit for human consumption, as disgusting body effluvia filled with chemicals and pus. They implicate milk in harmful capitalism, environmental degradation (cows require large amounts of water and they produce ozone-destroying methane gas), speciesism, and even racism. White nationalists use it as a symbol of racial purity; one rioter carrying a profascist flag at the April 15, 2017, "free speech" (really hate speech) rally in Berkeley, California, ostentatiously downed a quart of organic milk on camera before charging into battle.

These contentious meanings pass into breast milk. Jen, a prolific milk donor from Los Angeles, nursed her child "the same way I would make a point to buy my kid organic food. . . . I don't know how you can do one and not think the other matters." Milk is health. But she hesitated to give her son cow's milk when he got older, because as a "factory food," it seemed "far more bizarre than nursing."

Historical and social context always matter to the infant feeding experience. Oddly enough, while cow's milk has gained traction as a healthful drink and class marker in China, where an even greater proportion of the population is lactose intolerant, breastfeeding has fallen off.[48] Camille Li studies how formula—which can be purchased by urbanites with money but less so by the rural poor—has become de rigueur for middle-class aspirants, the opposite of what has been happening in the United States since the 1970s.[49]

Milk that some might call "pure" seems sterile to others. Valerie, an engineer, mother of four, and evangelical Christian, explained, "I have read things about milk banks that they are pasteurizing it, which, you know, kills some of the really, really good stuff in there and that they are reselling it to, like, these preemies; they are making some kind of milk product out of it for preemies in the hospital, and it is just kind of weird. It just doesn't seem natural, and I don't think anybody should have to pay for this milk."

A view of cow's milk as pasteurized, sterilized, homogenized—and white—makes it seem pure and safe. Breast milk, though, contains more enhancements: from antibodies to more ephemeral properties like maternal love. Flash pasteurization kills bacteria indiscriminately (whether harmful, innocuous, or beneficial) and weakens immunity-boosting molecules. Valerie and other milk-sharing parents preferred "fresh milk" from the source, they told me, over human milk that has been processed and repackaged into inert blandness in the name of safety. For them, richness overrides risk. And this intangible richness makes it morally wrong to "denature" the substance and then impassively sell it.

TROUBLING SITUATIONS

Caregivers get into exceptional breastfeeding for exceptional reasons. From medical events to divorce to financial problems, many unforeseen situations threaten breastfeeders' goals and otherwise change the breastfeeding relationship. Stress or illness may reduce milk supply, sometimes precipitously so. Returning to the paid workforce leads to myriad adjustments.

Caregivers end up cofeeding, using donor milk, and/or extending breast-feeding often as a response to particular situations that arise. They usually do not set out to be different. Instead, they constantly have to negotiate social pressure and internalized expectations about the "proper" course in raising infants and children.

Additional stigmas rear their ugly heads, along with a fresh crop of practical matters to figure out, like coordinating with others and managing the milk. Ariel ended up exclusively pumping because her daughter never developed an appropriate suck reflex after a traumatic birth. Ariel felt shame when she gave her daughter a bottle in public. She offered to tell me her story because she wanted other exclusive pumpers to read about it and feel less alone, less judged.

New role adjustments happen out of necessity. Kiki nursed her brother's one-year-old out of desperation when he would not stop screaming while she was babysitting him. This incident began a regular arrangement and fostered an ongoing mutual affection between Kiki and her nephew. Following an unexpected divorce and the start of a job that entailed long hours and a commute, Candace and her daughter sought solace and reconnection through their breastfeeding. They reversed the move toward weaning, and the girl ended up breastfeeding until age four. "I knew people thought it was strange, but I didn't really care," Candace told me.

"We will do whatever it takes to do it," said Dorinne about providing her adoptive children with breast milk in the face of opposition at the hospital. The same sentiment holds true for Sandra and her wife. In their case, it was emergency postpartum gallbladder surgery and a hungry baby that led them to get creative. When Sandra's milk supply plummeted, a close friend stepped in to offer pumped milk and to the nurse the baby. This seemingly strange innovation came at a social cost: it was a blow to the parents' perceived ability to provide. Sandra felt more worthy of help, though, by having tried everything, including "every supplement you can think of" to get the supply back. Medical sociologists call this the double bind, in which society expects someone with physical limitations, like an illness, to be proactive about their situation.[50] It is a moral imperative that mothers and others try to breastfeed through any problems. As Sandra asked rhetorically, what else were they supposed to do with a hungry baby? The preexisting intimacy with this "very, very, very good friend" who nursed their baby also helped make it OK. Sandra was subtly insisting that they had not strayed too far from normal.

I heard a number of stories of idiosyncratic events—not always fire engine emergencies—in which nursing someone else's baby just happened. Sabine and her best friend, both graduate students, fell to breastfeeding each other's children out of necessity while trading childcare and time for their thesis research. The friend's son was "pretty mommy attached" and would not take a bottle. Sabine explained, "I was OK with it, and she was OK with [it]. It seemed pretty normal." The arrangement was not something they needed to make a formal agreement about or even discuss at length. They just did it when the need presented itself.

Even though breastfeeders may become exceptional just by responding in seemingly ordinary ways to ordinary needs that arise, others (like family members, the public, and medical providers) may not easily accept it. They may want to enforce some boundaries around intimacy. It was not always a co-nursing utopia in Kiki's family. She recalled the following conversation that ensued when her cousin tried to surreptitiously give permission for Kiki to nurse the cousin's child while babysitting:

COUSIN: I guess if he fusses, do your thing.
COUSIN'S HUSBAND: What do you mean "your thing?"
COUSIN: Um, if he fusses.
HUSBAND: She should call us?
COUSIN: No, Kiki, just do your thing.
HUSBAND: No, no, no, that is just weird.
KIKI: OK. I'm out. I will call you if your baby cries. I don't want to be part of this discussion. [Laughing]

Kiki pointed out that the cousin kept calling breastfeeding "your thing" in hopes that the husband would not understand. It dawned on him what they were talking about, and he balked. This reaction made Kiki feel rejected. She told me, "I was like, 'Oh! Gross?!' [mimicking her cousin's husband]. You think I'm like, 'Oh look, your son is nursing? This is so exciting for me?'" Soon after the interaction, Kiki thought about it and felt offended, concluding that her male relative had sexualized her breasts and breastfeeding. But she did not try to change his mind, choosing instead to respect his right to set touch boundaries around his child. Her standpoint as an exceptional breastfeeder differs from that of the wider public, which is not particularly aware of breastfeeding diversity.

As Kiki discovered, people question breastfeeders' motivations when they diverge too much from the norm. Nursing a child as old as eight garners widespread disapproval even from the usual champions of breastfeeding. Are they a little touched in the head like various literary villains? Extended breastfeeding by the Game of Thrones character Lysa Arryn, portrayed as the creepiest helicopter mom ever, exploits this trope. But Lanie, the maverick lactation consultant and mother who calls skin-to-skin bottle-feeding "breastfeeding," nursed her daughter for that long. The child seemed to need it. Lanie followed her lead, putting off weaning as the child reached six, seven, and then eight years of age. She eventually discovered that her daughter suffered severe vision problems; the child was going blind day by day, and nursing helped her orient herself to the world around her. Just because exceptional breastfeeding becomes necessary does not mean it will be socially acceptable, however. The family's community rejected them despite the extenuating circumstances.

Latisha reflects on the dilemma of nursing in public versus respecting the black community's standards of modesty:

> There is just so much stigma around it in the African American community. Women are ridiculous. They kind of feel like you are being immodest. Like you are showing your breasts to show your breasts. But it is not a sex organ. It is an organ for feeding your baby, to nurse your baby. That is the misconception that we have in the African American community. That you shouldn't show your breasts. But if a woman walks out on stage with all of her breasts out because she is performing, that is completely normal. But for me to feed my baby, that is an issue. So it was very scary. But now I don't care what other people think. So I had to kind of check myself: "Why are you doing all this? Just feed your baby."

Latisha engaged in self-affirmation and deliberately chose to ignore the naysayers who would oppress her. But this resistance was "scary." And it upset Latisha that other women were in on this policing. Plenty of breastfeeders give up because of these pressures. Nursing in public may not seem like exceptional breastfeeding to some, but it is to Imani, also a black mother.

Her mother kept asking her why she would not give her baby a bottle since that would be more modest. Imani endured social isolation with her first child in order to avoid nursing in front of anyone. But when she had a second child, she breastfed in public in spite of her mother's views. It wasn't easy, but Imani began nursing everywhere, she said, to help others see that is normal for black women to breastfeed.

Exceptional breastfeeders deal with stigma, uneasy role adjustments, the double bind imperative to "try everything" normative first, and a drive to "do whatever it takes" to provide the benefits of breast milk or breastfeeding. (And sometimes, exceptional breastfeeding "just happens.") Powerful social forces push them into exceptional breastfeeding, and other social forces stigmatize them for it. Their family and friends, however, can make or break the experience.

INTIMATE JUDGMENT

"Oh, my God, is she still on the tit?" one of Lily's friends asked her, incredulous. Lily, a twenty-five-year-old single mother, constantly had to fend off these sorts of bald questions. The interrogations came from her on-again, off-again boyfriend, a police officer whom she described as politically conservative and a traditional guy; from her friends, none of whom were able to nurse their babies; and from her fellow social workers at the office, who did not understand why she still needed to slip away to pump several times per day. Lily explained that breastfeeding a baby more than a year old was simply unheard of in her social circles.

Her sisters and her mother had more up-to-date opinions, though. They thought everyone should try to breastfeed for the first weeks and months of the baby's life. During her pregnancy, Lily felt pressure from her family to commit to breastfeeding. She confided to me, "I always said, 'Yes, [I would breastfeed],' but in my head, I always thought, 'Oh, I'm not really going to.'"

She did after all. Her tiny daughter arrived too early and lived her first weeks in the NICU, confined to an incubator and hooked up to monitors. Lily, frustrated by this separation from her baby, turned to one of the powerful hospital-grade pumps populating the facility. She thought of the machine as a saving grace because it allowed her to provide some kind of material comfort for her infant. Other mothers who spent time in NICUs (like Eve, Susan, and Ariel) noted that pumping occupied them and gave them something useful to do when they could not hold their babies.

When it was finally time to take her baby home, breastfeeding turned out to be quite the puzzle, with eight perplexed lactation consultants trying to get the latch going, with cumbersome nipple shields to facilitate milk flow, and with lots and lots of tedious pumping. Lily continued breastfeeding in the absence of much social support; she sought out playgroups hosted by a clothing store and a diaper service just to be around other breastfeeding mothers. The internet helped her feel better about breastfeeding when she logged on to Human Milk for Human Babies (HM4HB). Lily felt guilty about forgoing the pump in favor of on-demand breastfeeding. She assuaged these feelings with pragmatism: "Hey, it's easier; it's portable." She asked anxiously, "She cries—how can I deny her?" But she also worried that she was not being charitable enough. If Lily could not find a comfortable narrative at any turn, it may be because others doubted her motivations.

Lily occupied multiple locations on the social spectrum of good and bad mothers. Policies and attitudes tend to put down mothers like her who are young, single, Mexican, and working class. But she has a college degree and a professional career. She knew that, depending on who was judging, she was a bootstrapping success story; a bit pretentious in her cosleeping, cloth diapering, breastfeeding ways; or a lamentable statistic. This swirl impacted her feelings and decision-making, but so did her baby's cry. The same friend who asked if the baby was "still on the tit" later told Lily that she was proud of her for breastfeeding.

Put that twee image of a loving mother gazing softly down at her blissful nursing infant out of your mind. Breastfeeding is almost never just mother and baby privately and symbiotically bonding. There is constant social negotiation with close family members and partners. Breastfeeders often are dealing less with impression management—wherein they present idealized versions of themselves to the public—and more with the entangled emotional, physical, and psychological needs of multiple individuals. While many of the exceptional breastfeeders I talked to recounted stories of tremendous intimate support for breastfeeding—lesbian couples sharing the breastfeeding duties, husbands providing "first aid" by suckling at the breast to unclog a troublesome duct, a grandmother pinch hitting by relactating to keep her daughters in school—just as often, these relatives interrupted the flow.

Roxanne's mother breastfed all five of her children; she was still "devoted to breastfeeding" decades later. But for this grandma, modesty was integral to righteousness. When the family hosted two Mormon missionaries at dinner, Roxanne nursed her baby at the table like always. Her mom, she said, "was just horrified and livid" and yanked Roxanne out of the room to chastise her in "hushed but very angry tones." When Roxanne balked at leaving dinner to nurse in private, her mother insisted, "No, you have to. I'm not going to have you nurse in front of these missionaries!" Roxanne stood up to her mother, and, like several of the women I interviewed, this mother and adult daughter continued to have periodic conflicts about breastfeeding decisions.

Clearly, breastfeeders' intimate associates use all sorts of undermining tactics from surreptitious formula feeding to snide comments and other emotional warfare—even outright fights—about the duration and frequency of nursing. Extended, or "longer-term," breastfeeding very frequently requires negotiation with the breastfeeders' partner, who may want more attention. Of course, sometimes the problem is just helplessness rather than any intentional resistance or withholding of support. When my first adoptive son arrived, I lactated spontaneously—becoming a mother was a joyous, emotional event that changed my body chemistry! But I had no idea how to breastfeed and my mother and husband could not help; I gave up within a day or two.

Given all the aforementioned struggles—the never-enough qualities of breast milk, various challenging life situations, and negative interventions from their closest loved ones—*why* do exceptional breastfeeders persist?

3 · THE MOTHER OF INVENTION

Persisting with Exceptional Breastfeeding

"Even just a little bit counted, and I was just bound and determined that even though I couldn't create a whole lot, that the little bit that I could create would be beneficial," insisted Mira. Why was she so "bound and determined" just to get her baby a little bit of her milk? Why are other exceptional breastfeeders willing to weather all the layers of trouble, from the social stigmas to internal doubts to practical and medical obstacles? The short answer is that there are extensive and distinct benefits to exceptional breastfeeding.

Exceptional breastfeeders may radically redefine breastfeeding. They create and perform an array of redemptive choices—coming up with ways to be successful at breastfeeding, "even if it's a cobbled together replacement for nursing a baby," as Ariel, an exclusive pumper, said. An ethnographic interview study of women's breastfeeding experiences in the United Kingdom identified four types of "moral work" in breastfeeding: biographical preservation, biographical repair, altruism, and political action.[1] These first two categories work well to explain the persistence of some exceptional breastfeeders. Breastfeeding can be "biographical preservation" as a way of proving one's self-concept as a worthy mother, and breastfeeding can be "biographical repair" in redeeming that status when it falters.

Some exceptional breastfeeders revel in breastfeeding's power to heal the wounds of disruption. Breastfeeding heals prior traumas and repairs damaged relationships. Often it is this sort of unforeseen benefit that motivates people to continue breastfeeding through hardships. Exceptional breastfeeders also gain mastery, amassing knowledge and honing new, rarefied skills that they are loath to give up too easily. They get satisfaction from being good at unique ways of breastfeeding and, therefore, good at mothering. One study found that when parents approach breastfeeding as a project, it helps them to manage all of its "contradictions."[2] One expects some challenges and a learning curve with any project.

How do exceptional breastfeeders persevere through the difficulties, which come in varying degrees? First, the mechanisms (how they do it) and the motives (why they do it) for persisting with exceptional breastfeeding are inextricable. I use the term *adaptive breastfeeding* to describe the creative solutions that breastfeeders resort to in order to give breast milk or to suckle a child at the breast. The broader descriptor, *exceptional*, describes these phenomena as well as other nonnormative practices like extended (longer-term) breastfeeding[3] or co-nursing. Adaptive breastfeeding often involves an aid like the breast pump or a supplemental nursing system (SNS). Similar to wearing glasses to improve sight or using a cane to help with mobility, these devices allow certain breastfeeders to participate much like any other breastfeeder. With help from a pump or an SNS, they are able to comply with nutritional and good mothering ideals by giving their baby breast milk, even if their babies struggle to latch or they cannot produce enough milk.

Exceptional breastfeeders usually have to manage negativity—their own and that of their intimates. Part of this management calls for them to curtail the self-surveillance that is usually all-encompassing. Instead, they employ intentional imprecision and resist the urge to micromanage the body, a liberating proposition. Exceptional breastfeeders have to constantly renegotiate their relationships with the nursling(s), their other children, and frequently, another parent. As the baby grows and as the circumstances change, the breastfeeder cannot make all the choices in some kind of individualistic vacuum. Breastfeeders engage in collaborative intimacies, in which layers of mutual physiological, practical, and culturally influenced adjustments keep happening. To be sure, these solutions do not always wholly satisfy, as Ariel remembered:

Seeing a rubber silicone nipple in her mouth, it was almost hurtful. It made me feel like my body was failing me. And I was failing her. I was one of those people who is pregnant who really looked forward to nursing, and I was like, "I'm going to nurse in public! And I'm not going to care." . . . I've gotten more used to it now. When I feed her, I snuggle her tight. I hold her as if she was nursing, and I put the bottle in her mouth, but it feels wrong. It just doesn't feel natural. But I mean, to me, I can't nurse her, but I can give her breast milk.

Ariel had to let go of her dream of breezy public breastfeeding, part of a self that she imagined would be so in love with breastfeeding that she would perform it defiantly if need be. Exclusive pumping was a barely passable consolation prize for her. Though she simulated breastfeeding by close snuggling and by providing the ultimate nutrition, the artificial feeling never really went away.

REDEMPTIVE CHOICES

Aaliyah nursed each of her five adoptive children with an SNS filled with either homemade coconut-based formula or with donated breast milk. The formula came from a special recipe she made based on her own careful research into the ingredients that growing babies need. It provided adequate nutrition, but she still wanted to breastfeed. One of her motivations with breastfeeding was redemption. She lamented that she did not get to bond with her children through pregnancy, and she told me that the disappointment compelled her to figure out a way to breastfeed, to experience the process of intimate attachment, to "bond" another way. Nursing helped her recoup some respect for her body and confirmed her status as her children's rightful mother.

For Sheila, breastfeeding was part and parcel of a "better adoption," which included skin-to-skin contact and baby-wearing as efforts to foster attachment. Much of the talk around the home birth movement is about achieving a "better birth," free of needless and sometimes harmful medical interventions, and instead giving birth surrounded by family (sometimes) and the comforts of home. And hospice care at the end of life promises a better death, preferably pain-free and at home. Similarly, a better adoption through breastfeeding is about family and intimacy. Sheila considered telling her daughter, "I wish I could also say I breastfed you like your brother." She reasoned that only then would her daughter understand how important she was to Sheila. Although Sheila did not get to make this redemptive choice herself, she advocated for others to do so, and she used her own imperfect experience as a cautionary tale.

A better adoption in this vein is not just mimicking "natural parenting" trends, enacting the sort of good parenting expected of the middle class. Adoption already "queers" motherhood or destabilizes foundational assumptions about what makes a mother.[4] Simulating "good mother" expectations by acting like normative, gestational mothers—such as by breastfeeding—may comfort the adoptive caregiver and be a declaration that they are no different. But there is more going on, and it has to do with the idea that adoptive children begin life at a deficit. The situation may seem dire. Child development experts say that adoptive babies are at risk of lifelong attachment disorders. "Bonding" practices are preventative treatment then. The adoptive parent—who usually receives in-depth training about attachment problems—accepts this responsibility. Breastfeeding can be a way to establish a strong commitment.[5] It is not all about the milk and its properties. Whether adoptive breastfeeders induce lactation, use an SNS, or simply comfort nurse, they show themselves to be open-minded, "independent free thinkers,"[6] who are willing to push boundaries for the sake of their children and for their own redemption.

In this way, they may prove to themselves and everyone else that they are just as good as other parents—if not better. When I was receiving mandatory training for prospective foster parents before my first son was born and placed with me, the trainers often noted, with unintentional irony, that "adoptive parents are a special breed." According to them, adoptive parents share a tendency to seek intervention for their children early and often. People enter parenthood, or add to our families, with intention and preparation (after all, there are relatively few "surprise" adoptions as compared to surprise pregnancies). Breastfeeding, for adoptive parents and some others (like parents via a surrogacy arrangement), can be a part of this ultraparenting.

Redemptive choices may attest to personal growth and one's dedication to social progress, similar to Reich's concept of "self-determined mothering."[7] For example, when her fellow churchgoers became offended by her nursing during services, Alice, a forty-two-year-old black woman from New Orleans, kept it up because she thought it was right. In this same period of time, she also breastfed her two daughters' babies so that her daughters could stay in school without giving up on breastfeeding. Alice cited the maxim paraphrased from a quote by Maya Angelou: "Know better, do better."[8] This became a mantra, reminding her to keep breastfeeding even when others tried to discourage her. Her mother took charge during her first birth in a hospital and assumed they would both be giving the baby formula in bottles. Alice's decision to override her mother was especially difficult because Alice's sister had just passed away suddenly. Their mother wanted to work through her grief by putting all her energy into caring for the new grandchild. Alice's early decision to breastfeed instead of bottle-feed preserved an exclusive dyad. Then the child grew up to have a baby of her own, and Alice stepped in to help nurse her own grandchild.

HEALING "THE WOUNDS OF DISRUPTION"

"It's what helped heal the wounds of the disruption, and I believe it was a big help in him healing from the trauma in his early life," said Lanie. She was talking about a mother whom she told to "energetically imagine" that the bottle she gave her baby was actually her breast. Margaret, a former foster mother and a pro bono lactation counselor told me that one of her chief concerns has been "how to make peace with not being able to feed your baby solely, exclusively, [and] how to maintain a long-term breastfeeding relationship." She wanted mothers to count any variation of breastfeeding as a success. Both Lanie and Margaret transgressed breastfeeding norms and suffered the social consequences: social workers removed Margaret's foster child from her home when they learned she had breastfed him, and Lanie lost her status as a La Leche League (LLL) leader because she failed to follow their doctrines. Having survived these tough spots and continued to breastfeed anyway, they later proselytized the healing power of breastfeeding.

It is the breastfeeder at the center of this healing process, though the child benefits too. Marnie, an adoptive breastfeeder, said, "I don't know if actually I buy into the primal wound theory. I think it is a little extreme, but in some ways, I just feel it comforts him. And for me, it makes me feel like I am being a good mom inasmuch as I can be in a physical way. I know I can be a good mom in an intellectual way and in an emotional way." She did not nurse her son to heal him from the loss of his birth mother. This rationale gets bandied about in adoptive breastfeeding circles, but I do not think it is the prime motivation to nurse one's adoptive or foster child. Marnie suckled her child to enact good mothering, to feel more thoroughly like a "good mom." It is part of the recovery for *her* loss in not having birthed him. Aaliyah's motivation was similar: "This might sound kind of selfish. I don't know that it was for the benefit of the baby. . . . It was a way of healing from the loss of the babies that I miscarried."

CURING THE BODY

There are many ways in which breastfeeding, loosely defined, heals. Healing can refer to the repair of social rifts, emotional or psychological pain, and physical and physiological ailments. Bailey dealt with her grief over her sister's untimely death by finding breast milk donations for the baby twins she left behind. Breastfeeding helped Tara, who identified as genderqueer (a nonbinary designation), process some of the dysmorphia she always had about her breasts. Carena's baby was born with serious medical problems, including a heart condition. For her, breastfeeding was "something I could do. That was the only thing. Because anybody could take care of your child, but only I could provide the breast milk." Being able to do something exclusive for him helped Carena cope. Foster and adoptive children who have gone through trauma (aside from the "primal wound" of being taken from their birth mothers), their new parents note, begin to heal more readily with breastfeeding—growing and thriving from the high-quality nutrition while simultaneously establishing strong social bonds.[9] Vanessa's daughter, who began nursing at age five, overcame severe attachment difficulties that resulted from previous abuse.

Breastfeeding heals in ways expected and unexpected. The medical community promotes breastfeeding as a way to help physically heal the postpartum body and help sick babies.[10] The benefits are well-rehearsed if not always thoroughly researched.[11] Yet it is breastfeeding's oft-unexpected healing power for the breastfeeders that helps motivate them to continue beyond normative boundaries:

We were naked, chest-to-chest all the time. And then the milk came in, and it was just glorious. Obviously, it's hurting because I was walking around topless all the time, and it changed everything for me about my breasts. Because our society sexualizes them so much. Then knowing that I wanted to breast-feed and not really knowing: the thing that really complicates it is that I was molested as a kid. There's stuff that goes with that and touch issues that come up, and I didn't have any of that. [Laughs] Once she was in the world, it was like, "This is right."

Tayshia initially felt torn about breastfeeding, both "knowing" that she wanted to do it and also "not knowing" if she could handle it given her past trauma. Breastfeeding could upset her emotional balance; the "boundaries of touch"[12] are carved more deeply in Tayshia's life. Popular culture, medical narratives, breastfeeders, and even well-meaning advocates frame breast-feeding as a depleting experience, to which writer Fiona Giles objects.[13] The breastfeeder gives up free time and loses sleep and energy. Several of my respondents complained that their breasts lost their "perkiness." At best, breastfeeding seems to be a process of reciprocal satisfaction for breast-feeder and nursling. Tayshia's early dread was more profound than the typi-cal worries about being depleted or not knowing how to breastfeed. It could reopen painful wounds. Her laughter noted in the above passage, however, indicates that something else happened. She found relief and joy in "glo-rious" breastfeeding, something she and her daughter, Zee, kept doing for years. Everything felt "right," and Tayshia's gratitude to Zee for her own healed trauma continues to this day, several years postweaning. Reflecting on breastfeeding, she gushed, "It nurtured her, and it nurtured me. . . . I love it!" Giles calls on everyone to start considering breastfeeding as a type of self-care rather than self-sacrifice.[14] Of course, this narrative only works if breastfeeders themselves control it!

ESCAPING BLAME

The healing power of breastfeeding overlaps with redemptive choices. Mira, mentioned above, explained:

[Breastfeeding] was very, very healing. Because the first time, not being able to give birth and not being able to breastfeed, was shot one and shot two. It was like, here is a woman; I am supposed to be able to do these two things. I have been told that my whole life. This is what everyone in the medical community tells me I am supposed to do, and yet I can't do either one. Had I been born one hundred years ago, me and my child would have died apparently. And so for me to have been able to give birth successfully and then to be able to have my baby at my breast—I knew that it wasn't my milk that he was having—but to have him there was extremely healing. To realize that it was my breast that calmed him down . . . it was just, for me, it was very, very healing to be able to do that the second time.

Mira experienced redemption and healing with a better birth and a better breastfeeding experience when her second child came along. She repeatedly said that having the child at her breast—regardless of the fact that she could not produce much milk—healed her from feelings of failure. Her body served her baby's needs—to "calm him down"—and this success comforted Mira. It was probably not only the "medical community" contributing to her idea that she was off-track as a mother and as a woman; Mira was also a former Mormon, raised with religious doctrine that reveres motherhood for women above all other life pursuits. (Roxanne, another ex-Mormon said that motherhood is "the exalted path, instead of priesthood for men.") In any case, Mira pushed past these implicit judgments and felt more fulfilled as a result.

Sometimes, subpar experiences with birth and breastfeeding are iatrogenic—that is, medical interventions introduce the problems in the first place.[15] But would-be breastfeeders suffering through failed attempts may internalize the blame. Ellen was in her early twenties when she had her first child at a hospital. She realized later that her medical team made all the wrong decisions, complicating her birth and impairing her ability to breast-feed. She cried constantly and she pumped every few hours to no avail. "I wasn't even getting a drop. I was completely dry," she said, recalling her devastation. After the first few days, she doubled her pumping frequency and mustered three ounces, all poured together, for one week's effort. See-ing that measly three ounces cut her deeply. Hours of near-incessant pump-ing each day for a week would fill a freezer in many cases. Through all of it, she demonstrated resilience, trying and trying to make breastfeeding work with little outside help. Against the odds, and with a stroke of luck, she says, her baby figured it out. A few years later, pregnant again, Ellen "[did her] research" and learned about home birth. She planned to breastfeed but

harbored great trepidation. Then this happened moments after her daughter's birth: "She just laid on my chest and bopped three times and landed
right on my nipple and started breastfeeding perfectly, immediately. And it
was really cool for me to see that after having a birth without medications
and [without] all these interventions and so much toll on my body and then
having Michaela's birth and just seeing her just slide right into breastfeeding so easy." This is a redemption story if there ever was one. With multiple
attempts to initiate breastfeeding, Ellen shifted the blame from herself to
the defeating circumstances of hospital birth. In our conversation, it became
clear that Ellen eventually concluded that she and her child were victims of
others' poor choices and a flawed system.

Many breastfeeders fare just fine initiating in hospitals, in spite of a
clinical environment that can sabotage breastfeeding as other research indicates.[16] But *exceptional* breastfeeders are likely to get that exceptional status
because they encounter trouble—sometimes iatrogenic trouble—and find
a way around it. Escaping blame also becomes a process of self-discovery.

Exceptional breastfeeders surprise themselves with their own resilience
and determination. Lanie's expansive notion of breastfeeding came from
lived experience: "I would hold him at home skin-to-skin, and I would even
pull my T-shirt up and put the bottle under and nurse him. And that's what
we called it. We called that nursing." For her, this "nursing" was a road to
self-discovery. The difficulties involved a rocky adoption process and creative feeding methods and a medically fragile infant. Her former friends' kids
would threaten their family's private narrative: "That's not nursing! That's a
bottle." The La Leche group she had been part of for many years could not
understand her feeding choices, and the members became unsupportive.
She said, "Because I breastfed Ella, it led me down this path. Of positive parenting and being connected to my children and also really creating myself,
which is a healing of me, I have to say." Lanie said breastfeeding helped heal
her own childhood trauma and that it led her to intense soul-searching.

Although pumping is a "second-best" way of getting the milk to one's
baby, it is a "compensatory act," through which breastfeeders can still enact
good mothering.[17] Milk donation compensates even more in ways that are
not only redemptive but also healing. Like most donations, it feels like a
good deed. Stella planned her pumping schedule for her pregnant friend
who had had a double mastectomy. Being able to help benefited Stella as
well as her friend who had survived cancer.

We cannot assume that the healing power of breastfeeding is universal or that everyone applies it in the same way. Aaliyah declined to make any connection between her own status as a breast cancer survivor and her intensive dedication to breastfeeding her adoptive children; all the women in her family had experienced breast cancer, so it seemed an almost normal part of life.

Eve's experience exemplifies unexpected healing. Tragically, Eve's baby died in the neonatal intensive care unit (NICU). She pumped her milk for donation. Lactating mothers who lose their infants usually receive advice for how to stop their milk supply, sometimes by binding their breasts or taking certain medications. Counselors often think of the milk-filled breast as an obvious physical reminder of loss and a source of emotional pain. But this experience does not hold true for everyone. When I signed permission for my father's organs to be donated after his sudden death, for example, something good came from tragedy and provided a measure of comfort. Being able to do something physically taxing and numbingly repetitive—pumping, in Eve's case—can also have a soothing effect. As far as I know, researchers are not systematically tracking the frequency of milk donation by mothers whose babies die in infancy, but the anecdotes are piling up on breastfeeding-related internet sites. Word is getting out about this option for dealing with grief.

A holistic redefinition of breastfeeding enhances its healing powers. Exceptional breastfeeders can have more ways to redeem their embodied identities as good and fit parents. This nuanced, uplifting discourse may well encourage nonnormative breastfeeding. These are transcendent transgressions.

MASTERY

More prosaic perhaps is the development of specialized skills and knowledge around extraordinary breastfeeding. "I want to donate. I feel like a pro at it!" Adriana, a mother of three, enthused. Mastery of various aspects of breastfeeding—and especially unusual ways to breastfeed—demonstrates parents' dedication and resourcefulness on behalf of their children. Margaret, now in her fifties, located a pump made from auto-industry parts and a baby food jar so she could earn a living and still breastfeed back in the 1980s before pumps improved. And because they also want to see some payoff for their investment of time, effort, and finances, breastfeeders may continue past their initial goals or past what is "necessary." Kris, a comother of two who struggled with breastfeeding for a long time, joked, "Fast-forward two years and I can nurse this kid upside down or in a bar!" These lay experts may value their knowledge for its exclusivity, morph into role models, or even become so used to their singular routines that they liken it to an addiction.

CONTRAPTION TALK

It was fun for me to engage in some mutual "contraption talk" with the breastfeeders I interviewed. I participated in online conversations in which I provided my takes on the different SNS devices available. One woman posted about the device I liked: "It saved our breastfeeding relationship!" We get used to thinking that technology distances us from one another, but in her case, it had the opposite effect.

Like all gearheads and gadget geeks, breastfeeders like to share their hacks, but sometimes the rigs are just frustrating. For example, Amy, a mom of two, fumbled with and eventually rejected the sorry excuse for an SNS that her lactation consultant gave her to try. I get it: I once gleefully threw my Medela-brand SNS in the trash. The mother-invented Lact-Aid, which I ordered from an elderly woman over the phone since they were not yet sold online, was much better. I no longer had to sit up ramrod straight to feed Leo; I could doze off, reclined, as he nursed intermittently as babies do.

Contraptions can be lifesavers, according to breastfeeders like Adriana, whose baby could not take formula or the breast; she used a nipple shield, meant to be a temporary aid for babies with poor latch ability to get milk at the nipple and stay at the breast. Stella related this story: "An IBCLC [International Board Certified Lactation Consultant] said, 'What you need are nipple shells.' I was [like], 'Nipple shields?' I said, 'They had me using these nipple *shields* to give me something to get her to attach to,' and she said, 'No, no, you need shells.'" Stella needed this unusual fix to support her large breasts for nursing. She said that after she put these "little plastic things in [her] bra," her daughter "latched on and never looked back." She only used them once but credited them for her breastfeeding success.

Contraption talk can highlight inventiveness, but sometimes it's about shopping. In my field notes at a breastfeeding support group, I recorded:

> There's a mom with no makeup, wearing her hair in a ponytail, dressed in floral leggings and a tank top sitting on the floor nursing her three-month-old (she tells the volunteer who checked us in the baby's age). There are many colorfully patterned accoutrements on a blanket on the floor in front of her "station": additional blankets, a changing pad, fashionable diaper bag, water bottle, a Sophie the Giraffe toy. She talks mainly to her onesie-wearing baby, but I think we are meant to hear. "You aren't getting much, are you?" she coos. "I just pumped this side, that's why." In between checking her phone, she says, "Are you feeling better now?" "Feeling happy?" "Are you ready to get weighed?"

Upon arrival, each of the other moms (except one, who was more than an hour late for the hour-and-a-half-long session), wearing the same basic uniform, spread out a blanket and all her stuff in a similar manner to the first mom before taking her baby out of a car seat. They asked questions, and Rose, the lactation consultant, provided all sorts of practical advice about timing feedings and the like. But mostly they talked about commercially available products: wearing "lily pad" breast pads to a wedding, "mastering" the bottle warmer, effectiveness of "ice pack bottles" in extending milk's freshness, where to buy the slowest flow nipples, visiting the lactation store to fit the correct bottle nipple rings, best types of infant carriers for dads to "give mom a break," the importance of having a "pumping bra," the trickiness of sanitizing a secondhand pump, and investing in extra bottles and "extra pump pieces."

Consumerism shapes our lives and our aspirations. Barbara Katz Rothman writes, "Birth and food, once so profoundly part of women's worlds of production, ultimately came to be acts of consumption, all about intelligent, thoughtful, careful shopping, and making good choices."[18] This pattern holds true for breastfeeding, which is both part of our procreative lives and part of feeding our children. Shopping for breastfeeding products helps shape motherhood by providing a way to express diligence, caring, and sacrifice.[19] Breastfeeders' careful selection of the right products, their "informed consumption,"[20] is part of their work as good mothers/caregivers. It is also a way to assert class status. Exceptional breastfeeders often extend this dynamic further because they have to fill niche needs and because it feels like their motherhood fitness is in doubt. The existence of adaptive devices also helps normalize adaptive breastfeeding—there would be no SNS to buy if others did not also need it.

Rose and I grabbed lunch after one of the sessions, and I asked her how she got into her work. She told me that when she started a couple of decades earlier—she had been an obstetric nurse—it became clear that local mothers did not know where to buy breastfeeding supplies like nursing pillows and nursing bras. Rose started selling the products at the hospital, which later built a birthing center (for those with good insurance coverage), and that venture grew into lactation consulting. The services are free; the products are not. At least initially, the sales helped justify and support the lactation counseling services.

The financial investment in all these supplies probably induces breastfeeders to use them—many of them purchase deep freezers, predicting that they will one day be full of pumped milk. Still, not all breastfeeding stuff gets put to use. Everyone I know who bought a "Boppy" or "Brest Friend" nursing pillow ended up using them for other purposes, if at all. And even though the products are available, I could not find any cisgender men who actually used one of the jokey "daddy devices" in which a harness with nipple-topped bottles is worn over the chest (I did talk to men who thought about it, and I saw an internet pic of a dad from Port Saint Lucie, Florida, who poked a bottle through his shirt to feed with). Nevertheless, we can all imagine such a scenario thanks to the scene from the comedy *Meet the Fockers* in which actor Robert DeNiro wears a "manary gland" for laughs as an oddball doting grandfather.

Getting good with the tools permits ever more creative applications and flexibility. Better pumps not only help keep women at their paid jobs but also allow for milk sharing, which leads to all sorts of novel arrangements. For cofeeding couple Sandra and Tara, contraption talk from a local breastfeeding group, such as discussions about different sized flanges to make pumping go better, supported their ability to continue making enough milk for their baby.

In a prime example of our ongoing "cyborgification,"[21] the parts become a part of our bodies and of our relationships. My own son took in a tube along with my nipple as he swallowed milk from my body that was mixed with donor milk from the bag around my neck. This integration can be made even more sci-fi with the addition of milk-tracking apps and the like; alternatively, we can experience it as homespun DIY inventiveness.

INNOVATING PROTOCOLS

Adaptive breastfeeders have to figure out how to apply the available technologies given their own circumstances. I attempted to classify all the different protocols I learned about in the eighty-three interviews, coming up with protocols for pumping; inducing lactation; stemming the flow; increasing the supply; weaning; stopping lactation; acquiring and ingesting lactogenic foods, herbs, and medications; milk storing; milk sharing; milk packing and shipping; selecting milk recipients; soliciting milk donations; cofeeding; mixed feeding; supplementing; extended nursing; treating jaundice; and maintaining breastfeeding tools (e.g., pumps, bottles, SNSs). Getting a system in place and making a routine seem necessary for success, and any hitch can lead to problems in reaching breastfeeding goals. Those who find a comfortable rhythm usually attribute their success to flexibility. Whether they try another tool or feeding pattern or whether they change the way they frame success, some exceptional breastfeeders begin to approach breastfeeding as a "journey" rather than a specific set of milestones. All the attention to detail makes this an easier proposition. A dozen interviewees told me that they take breastfeeding day by day. All breastfeeders have to adapt to their babies changing rapidly and their milk supplies fluctuating, but some exceptional breastfeeders feel fortunate to be able to breastfeed at all.

Figuring out the pumping protocol is the key to much of exceptional breastfeeding. Some frequent breast pumpers I talked to described pumping as a "respite" or "relaxing" in its monotony. More often, pumpers felt ambivalent. Ariel, talking about pumping, said, "I would have quit in the beginning because I was so exhausted. . . . It's not a fun thing to be doing. When you are nursing a baby, you can snuggle with them and look at them and kind of touch their skin. But then you are sitting next to a big machine that makes weird noises, and it is not physically very comfortable."

Pumping, for her, was "tedious." Ariel "thought about quitting every single day" because of the endless cycle of "feed, pump, feed, pump, feed, pump," but she did it because she wanted her baby to have the "best." She became proud of her resilience and the happy consequences of all that pumping: her child stayed off formula, and she donated large amounts of milk to others in need. Mira, by contrast, got little from the pump in terms of milk or in feelings of success. But her mastery of the SNS instead allowed her to position herself as successful in a different realm. For Ariel, mastery meant producing breast milk given exclusively in a bottle. For Mira, it meant the opposite: bonding by suckling in the absence of milk production.

Susan had some initial "supply issues" that she soon resolved. Maybe because she did not have to contend with the kind of major barriers that Ariel and Mira faced, she approached protocol development more play-fully: "I like having my hands free. So I'll get it all hooked up in the car and then have the nursing cover over the top. If I get pulled over, I won't freak the cop out or be flashing any truck drivers. I let it run while I'm driving. I can turn it off while I am driving easily by just pulling the tubing out."

She invented this pumping protocol to allow her to produce and donate as much as possible while also breastfeeding her children up to age three and volunteering with LLL, a big part of her life. She also demonstrated her mastery over breastfeeding by managing her milk for different recipients. She separated milk that she pumped while taking ibuprofen—that was for informal donations—from unadulterated milk destined for the milk bank. Susan avoided medications, "strictly" followed the milk bank guidelines that limit caffeine and alcohol, rented a high-quality breast pump at her own expense, and required her family to accommodate the "big blocks of time" she set aside for pumping at home. This commitment allowed her to reach a rewarding level of proficiency: "[I donate] to help these critically ill infants who need this milk, but also I think I've enjoyed kind of raising the bar and making it seem more normal for other people. . . . By making this trail a little bit more worn, the other women who find comfort in this area, will not feel so alone doing the same thing. . . . I also like the idea of, 'Oooh, maybe I could kind of break some records?' That would be fun."

Susan, careful not to seem too competitive or self-aggrandizing, also indicated that she would not negatively judge anyone who did not donate and that she knew of donation records that could never be beat. She could not quite bear to call herself an inspiration, but she meant for her mastery over milk producing to be just that. Innovative protocols become a personal investment that breastfeeders do not want to see go to waste by ending their participation prematurely.

HABITS

"People are relying on this milk, and I've been supplying milk, and how do you just stop?" asked Lily. Lily separated breastfeeding and pumping, realizing that she could just feed her daughter on demand and not pump so much for others. Cutting off production, though, can be a difficult choice to make for many milk donors. Some creative breastfeeders have to adjust their lives dramatically to accommodate the protocols they put in place. As a consequence of this painstaking success, their end goals may get blurry. "Why not see what the ol' body can do?" asked Sparrow, a transfeminine breastfeeder interviewed on the *Breastfeeding Outside the Box* podcast.

And even though they know that breastfeeding is a discrete time in their lives, they may be reluctant to stop because they are enjoying some of the unanticipated benefits.[22] Susan explicitly connected continued breastfeeding and pumping with her own well-being:

> I will just sit down at a pump, and by the time I am done and I get up, I feel better again. That's part of why I have stuck with it: I just think it does help me feel better. I think it helps my body. You know our bodies are designed to lactate. I think the ways our bodies are programmed, women are supposed to be lactating for years, and so I didn't want to take that away from body. And I think it's made it easier for me despite the intense time; there have been issues as far as working and the pumping. I think it's been easier on my body, which has been easier on my emotions, just to keep my hormones where they're supposed to be.

Susan persisted with pumping not just for altruistic reasons but for herself. It felt so good that it was worthwhile even though it was hard to pump around her work schedule. Despite the essentialist rationale she provides, Susan was not just fulfilling her biological destiny but borrowing from the narrative that female bodies are designed to lactate for years as a "cultural logic"[23] that could fortify her choices as the right ones. The society in which she lives does not typically support the choice to breastfeed (and pump) for years on end. Medical advice tends toward the "dosage" mind-set. Babies should breastfeed exclusively for six months and then breastfeed along with supplemental foods for one year or maybe two. Breastfeeders who exceed this prescription feel pressure to explain themselves. More pointedly, Susan nursed her children for a long time and donated her milk (very selectively) as an important part of her life, as a healthful practice, and as a therapeutic measure. Her pleasure in it was not a comfortable enough explanation. She also has to be seen as complying with the contemporary edict that all of our behaviors should be useful and healthful.

It is not just the babies and toddlers who have a hard time with weaning but the breastfeeders too. Kadijah remembered:

> It was bittersweet. Because I felt like, while I was nursing, there was the useful-ness going on with my breasts. Like they had this really strong purpose, and it became part of my daily life, just part of my rhythm, using them in some sort of way that was beneficial to my child. And I noticed as we got closer and closer to the time where we were not going to nurse anymore that I started to gain weight. Maybe that is a little vain. [Laughs] I was like, "Don't stop!" . . . I was hoping there was somebody who needed me to feed their baby or something.

She savored the sense of purpose that she got with breastfeeding and the rhythmic routine it brought. Kadijah felt the change in her body as the energy output decreased, and it took a while to accept that change. She did end up relactating for a friend suffering from severe postpartum depres-sion; the baby lived with Kadijah for weeks. "I would've done it one million times," she said. Unlike some of the others I interviewed, it was not hard-won exceptional breastfeeding that accounted for her enthusiasm. Breast-feeding was easy for Kadijah from the start. Rather, the ease of and love of breastfeeding led her to exceptional breastfeeding; she nursed others' babies to keep the experience going. Plus, she liked the way it slowed her weight gain. Partly because of the limits of expert advice and partly because of the other demands on breastfeeders, many of them overlook this lack of a hard stop to breastfeeding as a viable option. Yet some breastfeeders may appreciate a gentle weaning for themselves, not just for their babies.

EXTRALOCAL KNOWLEDGE

"Doing the research," as Tayshia called it, is an integral part of pregnancy, childbirth, and breastfeeding for many American women.[24] There are myr-iad options and personal decisions to be made. Women read everything they can and plan, plan, plan (and buy all the stuff). *What to Expect When You're Expecting* and *The Womanly Art of Breastfeeding* are modern classics—that is, for white, middle-class women. There are now more resources—books, blogs, and online groups—that specifically cater to women of color and to queer parents. Some of the black women I interviewed credited the book *Birthing Justice: Black Women, Pregnancy, and Childbirth*, which takes an expansive, historic view and combines activism, scholarship, and personal perspectives, for opening their eyes and supporting their procreative resistance.[25] Seminars, pamphlets, and programs sponsored by the Women, Infants, and Children Food and Nutrition Service (WIC) and school-based initiatives promote breastfeeding among parents with fewer economic means. These days, the internet houses more information than any of us can handle. It is also very effective for spreading the word on exceptional varieties of breastfeeding.

And yet information is not neutral. One same-sex couple—who decided not to be interviewed at length—felt pressured to breastfeed by the queer community they encountered online and in person. One member of the couple first contacted me when someone posted my call for participants online because they wanted to let me know of their good reasons to bottle-feed with formula. All the online talk promoting queer couples' cofeeding made them uneasy and even a bit angry. In their case, the information comes with judgmental strings attached.

Sometimes exceptional breastfeeding practices need to be kept under wraps, meted out with purpose to a select few—leaving out meddling social workers (in the case of foster breastfeeding) or the too-curious public. "I nursed my daughter in public for nine or ten months, but because she was black and I'm white, there were way too many people way too interested, and I thought, 'I'm drawing attention to her that I don't think she needs,'" remembered Lisette. But at the same time, prospective breastfeeders need information and peer support. "Secret groups" on Facebook can be particularly helpful, but they still require vigilant moderating.

Transfeminine breastfeeders have few supports, and they worry about being open about it in public and online. Their breastfeeding attracts unwanted fetishists—or worse, outright vilification and harassment from internet trolls. Many trans people tire of being seen as research subjects or fodder for salacious headlines. Still, three interviews published on the internet—two on MilkJunkies.net, primarily a resource for transmasculine chestfeeders, and one from the podcast *Breastfeeding outside the Box*—provide personal stories and practical advice for transfeminine breastfeeders. As one mother, Sparrow, said on the podcast, "I want to [breastfeed] for [my son], and I want to do this for me . . . and for other transfeminine people so that they can see that it's possible. I felt like I had something to prove." This last reason compelled her to share her special, experiential knowledge about how to breastfeed and what it was like for her.

Like a knowing glance between friends, sometimes it is fun to harbor special knowledge and to feel like an iconoclast: "I feel quite smug if you really want the truth," Harriet confessed, talking about her "working breasts," the source of many donations and wet-nursing arrangements. Kris and Rachel learned how to produce and handle quality milk in such a way that "everybody knows that it is liquid gold when we deliver it." They became members of a veritable private club, working together to support other parents and other babies. Their offhand way of talking about milk and breastfeeding revealed playfulness and a level of comfort with their unique arrangement. Shawn, a breastfeeding lesbian mother who described her gender identity as "boyish," said of her milk, "I put it on this little spot! [Indicates spot on her face] And in [her] eyes when she got pink eye. We kind of just for the heck of it squirt it on whatever. I tried [it] in coffee. It is not yummy. It is not good—in coffee." Shawn felt slightly bewildered by the gender incongruity of producing milk with her masculine body, but she had fun with the milk. Some exceptional breastfeeders persist through all the stigma and practical difficulty in part because they enjoy having specialized knowledge and because they delight in their unique practices.

MANAGING NEGATIVITY

"What on earth were you doing in the car?" asked Marilyn's mother. Marilyn's choice to breastfeed each of her three children past the age of one became a big joke in her family, who had not heard of such a thing. They warned that she would be breastfeeding her son until he was eight and that she would have to run the bases with him when he played T-ball. She explained what she was doing while riding in a car in front of her parents' car: "I was trying to figure out how to nurse him while they were driving, so I didn't have to stop. I tried all sorts of weird positions that they could see through the window. I was kind hanging over the basket." Her mom asked pointedly, "Wouldn't it have just been easier to make him a bottle?" Her mother also cajoled her, "You know, you are just so tired. Don't you get tired of him tugging at you?" Marilyn said, "No," and her mother replied, "OK then," and let it go.

Having to deal with the negative judgments, disapproving looks, comments, and general puzzlement from family members and others may actually drive some exceptional breastfeeders' persistence. Like the middle-class white mothers Reich interviewed, some see breastfeeding as "social activism" and as an opportunity for "public education."[26] Sometimes this activism happens quite locally—in the car or at the dinner table. Roxanne declared herself an independent adult and the rightful decision-maker regarding her own children after having the fight with her mother (mentioned in chapter 2) over nursing in front of visiting young Mormon men. She educated her mother while also rebelling against her.

Yesenia managed her "macho cop" husband's distaste for extended breastfeeding—she nursed her three-and-a-half-year-old—by hiding it from him. She also worked in law enforcement, though in the office and not in the field. Since she already felt like the strange one for breastfeeding (most cops she knew could not breastfeed and still do their jobs), she figured she might as well go all the way with it.

Another motive/strategy for continuing with exceptional breastfeeding despite negativity is to "radiate confidence," as Katie described it. Vanessa, breastfeeding her adoptive children, stopped naysayers in their tracks: "Maybe I seemed competent, and they were not prepared to actually say anything because it was too shocking." Olivia, also a breastfeeding adoptive mother, voiced what several of the breastfeeders I interviewed said: "I tend to have an attitude that doesn't welcome any feedback." She thought perhaps her punk-rock look may have scared off any would-be critics in her conservative Texas hometown.

Others have to seek like-minded support in the face of negativity, either with online communities or by making new connections in real life. Sometimes people already in their lives who failed to support them at first come around. When Lily's once-discouraging friend finally offered her approval for Lily's decisions to breastfeed for a long time and to donate her milk, the two cried together. This long-withheld support gave Lily "the juice" to keep going.

Jeff, a gay father, and his partner hired a surrogate to bear their baby. He surrounded himself, fortress-like, with supportive people. This insulating strategy may be integral to the well-being of many queer parents. But he recounted a Facebook clash with a woman who "went on blast" about the "wrongness" of gay fathers' receiving donor milk. Jeff's mother came to his defense and shut the critic down, an incident that made him feel "hugely supported." He already trusted his mother's unconditional support, but her public advocacy on his behalf was a pleasant surprise that hardened his resolve to keep getting breast milk for his child.

Sometimes exceptional breastfeeders dismiss others' negativity as coming from a place of ignorance or misplaced authority. For example, Kendra breastfed her toddlers in spite of the father's and grandfather's insistence that breastfeeding "keeps them a baby" for far too long. Her divorce made it both easier and harder to do. She could breastfeed without interference in the moment, but shared custody undercut her milk supply (she had to pump frequently to keep any milk flowing after several days apart from her younger child, who was nursing at nineteen months—happily, the child told me during my interview with her mom).

Connie, a lesbian mother and marketing executive from Colorado who received donated milk for her child, said, "My sister is one of the only people in the world who will be completely frank with me, and she kind of wrinkled up her nose and said, 'You are giving him someone else's milk.'" Connie said, "Yes," and her sister responded "Oh, OK," waited a beat, and innocently asked, "Is that weird?" Connie's response—a frequent refrain among breastfeeders—was "We drink cow's milk, and at least . . . [the donor is] a human." She said, "My mum did the whole kind of pursed lips, 'Hmmm, interesting.'" Letting "pursed lips" negativity slide allows everyone to suspend judgment and keep the peace. Many family members and close friends begin to accept seemingly strange variations on breastfeeding when they see it working and the baby thriving. Alice, the breastfeeding grandmother mentioned earlier, was of two minds about it all. Breastfeeding, she decided, is the future of mothering for black women, and it was certainly right for her and her daughters. She persisted even though support was insufficient "because in our family and also in our culture, breastfeeding was not something that was done." She could not decide whether to include pictures or not in an article she wrote about grandmothers co-nursing:

I don't think my husband is comfortable. Because once I post the article, a lot of our friends, his family, his friends, his male friends, will see it. I don't know if he is comfortable, because this is all new to him. The whole process. Natural birth, natural childbirth, breastfeeding, all of this is just new, so he is getting comfortable with things, and I don't want to push it by putting too much on him. So I haven't gotten to that point, but I love women that are. I love seeing pictures of women that are nursing in public and are not covered. So it is kind of ironic that I love seeing it, but I haven't gotten to the place where I have gotten comfortable with it.

Alice used a cover while breastfeeding to ease the men in her family, particularly her spouse, into this new world of black women breastfeeding. Yet ironically, she did not hold others to that same standard of modesty. In a tightrope walk, she accommodated others' sensitivities while also pushing boundaries. Alice and others persist with breastfeeding outside of the norm to broaden people's attitudes—from the family to the community to the public at large. Although they often exercise discretion in strategic ways, others' negativity can be an incentive for exceptional breastfeeders to keep it up. Their continued breastfeeding actively resists the implication that what they choose to do is wrong somehow.

INTENTIONAL IMPRECISION

"I don't keep track. If you want to make yourself crazy as the mother of a newborn, count how many times a night they wake up and how many times a day they nurse," advised Sabine, a teacher and mother of two. Sometimes experienced breastfeeders purposefully give up on the measurement and counting and keeping track that are so much a part of the contemporary breastfeeding experience. Francine breastfed fourteen children—some she gave birth to and some she and her husband adopted. And yet she never pumped her milk and only gave formula to one child who required a feeding tube. "To me, it is just common sense that you are doing something naturally. As long as there is no emergency, it is just going to make sense. Our bodies are used to having babies. We produce milk. Babies eat milk," she maintained. The attitude is like that of someone who eats when they are hungry and declines to count calories. Francine, and others like her, free themselves from anxiety by minimizing their self-surveillance.

There can be negative consequences, however, if the casual approach also bypasses self-care. Kiki, who breastfed all eight of her children, never worried about how much she was producing or how much her babies were getting. She said with surprising nonchalance, "Recently, I've noticed, 'Oh, well. I am missing some teeth. They need some attention.'" Counter to the mainstream narrative, Kiki did not view breastfeeding as a maternal sacrifice. Kiki thinks she is generally healthy and worries little about herself, but she admitted to feeling depleted: "While my spirit has been having a great time, my body has been like, 'Whoa!' It is feeling a little bit neglected."

Some exceptional breastfeeders approach life's obstacles with more humor and ease than others (and, of course, some have more financial and social capital to ride out the hard times). Olivia needed donated milk for her first child, who she adopted, but produced plenty for her second child, who she conceived with the help of fertility treatments. She did not seek the optimal experience, unlike many normative breastfeeders. Whereas other recipients of donated milk feel apprehensive about their supply stores, Olivia wondered aloud how much milk it was and then flatly concluded, "It was enough." Pumping did not go well for her, and since her second infant thrived at the breast, Olivia declined to set aside a freezer stash and refused to add any unnecessary record-keeping tasks to her already busy life.

Still, Olivia went to great lengths to provide breast milk. She had to deal with customs agents when she took some across international borders between the United States and Guatemala. And amusingly, she attracted a curious crowd of indigenous women, who brazenly reached into Olivia's blouse to discover the SNS that allowed this *gringa* to nurse her adoptive Guatemalan daughter. She also had to cope with the shock—and material reality—of her husband leaving her while he was still in the throes of a long affair. Basically, she said, he had a second family. Through it all, she laughed off absurd situations and reckoned that precise attention to the minutiae of breastfeeding served no purpose as long as her children were doing well. Breastfeeding seemed to be an adventure to Olivia.

Dorinne, a nurse and adoptive mother of three who received donated milk, never paid "close attention" to the amount she received because she sustained a strong network of donors. She felt certain enough that she would never have to turn to formula, so she saw no reason to get "too obsessed." She was fully aware that other adoptive mothers worried themselves silly over it. Dorinne made a concerted effort to be satisfied with the knowledge that her children suckled at the breast, they got breast milk and not formula, and they got at least some of her milk. She did not need to go all out in an effort to boost the increments coming from her own breast when she could already check off all of her goals. She relied on her community to come through for her.

The intentional imprecision strategy runs counter to entrenched cultural norms that scientize food (measurement in cooking and counting calories train us for measuring and storing milk) and medicalize and monitor the female body.[27] Some self-identified "birth geeks," activist-practitioners in the birth world, advocate a more naturalistic approach to all birth- and infant-related endeavors. There is a hierarchy of the natural in this framing: unassisted home birth and direct-from-the-breast nursing are at the top and planned hospital C-sections and formula-filled bottle-feeding are at the bottom. The exceptional breastfeeders that I present in this book tend to fall somewhere in the middle, striving for natural but usually getting really precise about it. Those who take a more laissez-faire approach may have an easier time persisting with breastfeeding than those obediently "watching the line."

There is a privilege in being able to eschew worries about breastfeeding. First, a breastfeeder who can afford to be at home or who has a flexible paid job may be more able to forgo the pump altogether. Those without that luxury have to worry more about how much they produce and whether it is enough for their babies to get through the day with their hunger satisfied. Second, strong support networks and cultural capital matter. If a well-off mom in need of milk seeks some through her Facebook connections, she is now quite likely to get it from someone her real-life friends can vouch for. A gay dad may get flamed. Third, for a host of reasons already covered, some bodies cannot produce sufficient breast milk and some dyads cannot get breastfeeding going easily. They need to work at it, which often leads to a need to track the progress so that they can pinpoint where adjustments should be made.

Notwithstanding all these important variations in circumstance, there may be a lesson here. The conscious refusal to be meticulous and exact—sometimes this means sliding the goal a bit further from the natural ideal—and choosing instead to have a modicum of faith in one's efforts helps many a creative breastfeeder persist through the tough times long enough to reap the many benefits.

COLLABORATIVE INTIMACIES

A toddler quoted in an article by Karleen Gribble provided this reason for breastfeeding: "Because I love you, because I love breast milk."[28] In her unique work exploring children's perceptions of breastfeeding, Gribble finds that those who continued to nurse after having acquired language describe it as normal (of course!) and as having the following meanings: pleasure, delicious food, comfort and calming, emotional security, and closeness and intimacy.[29] Obviously, breastfeeding is always an "interembodied" experience.[30] There are always social dimensions as well as intra-actions. This mutual interdependency includes preverbal communications that range from the anatomical and physiological to the cues that babies give the caregiver and the cues that caregivers give the children. For example, Kiki said, "With each child—How do I say this? Their mouths are different. They just do it different. Plus my boobs change with every child. [Laughs] It is not quite the same, so we have to relearn the pattern for that child specifically and how they do it." As a result of each child having different needs and qualities and the breastfeeders' bodies and circumstances changing, weaning happens at different ages.

I was heartbroken when my son weaned himself at eleven months. After having gone to so much trouble to breastfeed and to bring in a milk supply, I fully expected to keep it up for at least a couple of years. He had other plans. This sort of asymmetry in weaning—often it is the breastfeeder who wants "her body back" before the child is quite ready—is typical. Either party may exercise veto power. The breastfeeder can stop offering the breast, or the child can take a permanent "nursing strike."

It also goes beyond dyad decisions. Sometimes the needs and desires of siblings come into the mix. Many breastfeeding children stop nursing when their mother becomes pregnant—the milk supply drops and the taste changes—but some pick it back up after the baby is born. Jessica nursed her daughter in stops and starts. She acquired an SNS and donor milk when her milk dried up during her third pregnancy so that she could keep her daughter at the breast. This worked for five months, and then the child went a year before starting up again. Jessica said, "I always find it funny that I can tell [friends] that this is the first time that I've ever nursed a child this age, but I've nursed a child who was older. Which is kind of weird if you think about it. It was kind of cool." Her pregnancy had been a surprise, and she explained her joy in being able to start again with the older child: "I felt like I had cheated her out of that time and out of that relationship with me." Jessica ended up negotiating with her almost two-year-old child to work out a comfortable way to tandem feed (the gentleness of the infant and the vigor of the toddler were difficult for her to take at one time). Her daughter "patiently wait[ed] her turn" until her younger brother's nursing session was done.

Tandem nursing breastfeeders who adjust to make room for their children to continue or restart breastfeeding not only maintain the dyad relationship but also expand it to include siblings. Lonny explained:

I think it really helped with the girls' bonding. [My first daughter] was three when [the second] was born. People had said that that could be a difficult age with the adjustment, but she has never had any jealousy or problem with her sister, and I think it was because she never felt rejected by her, and she always knew [the baby sister] will have first go. In the early days, [the older daughter] didn't feed much. She picked it up again later for some reason. I would feed the baby first, and then I would feed her until I [got] the hang of doing them both together.

Her older child—four at the time of the interview—stroked her baby sister's hair and feet a bit as they both nursed. The sisters also made eye contact with one another while breastfeeding. Her older daughter felt soothed— I witnessed her arrive home from kindergarten, jump into her mom's lap, and begin nursing as a way to reconnect after having been apart—and it helped Lonny's milk supply. The older sister played a role in producing milk for her sister. While convenient for Lonny, it was not the perfect arrangement. She had to adjust her technique (pacing and position) so the fast milk flow did not choke the infant. All three of them collectively persisted with breastfeeding because they enjoyed the intimacy.

Collaborative intimacy is tantamount to cofeeding families. Jeri and Allie both nursed their daughter, and they found that they needed to coordinate so that the baby had enough milk and they maintained appropriate milk supplies. Allie shared, "We just had to work it out schedule-wise. But then it ended up that I usually nursed her once a day, and then Jeri would do the rest, and then I would pump and freeze whatever else I had." The problem with that arrangement was that Allie's abundant supply led to painful engorgement. They decided to have Allie do most of the breastfeeding. Jeri, the egg donor but not the gestational mother, would step in for some special time with her daughter just once per day. This time block also provided her wife a welcome respite. They both pumped the excess for donation.

Another couple, Kelly and Marybeth, both induced lactation prior to even being placed on their adoption agency's list of waiting families. In a way, they began the breastfeeding relationship before their son even arrived: "We continued to pump, froze the milk, and just pumped. We were pumping fiends. We would do it at one o'clock in the morning—maybe it was later than that, maybe two o'clock or sometime in the middle of the night that they say that your milk sort of reaches a peak, so it is a good time to pump."

The support they gave each other—especially sharing nighttime feeding in the early months—made breastfeeding pretty easy, they said, and they kept it up until their son turned four. They initiated breastfeeding mainly because they wanted the closeness, but they continued for additional reasons: it is calmed their active son and had a therapeutic effect on his allergies.

Compromise and adjustment foster collaborative intimacies. For breastfeeding to continue being part of a positive relationship, breastfeeder(s), baby, and supportive family members have to balance one another's needs and capacities. Gwendolyn tandem nursed for a year but began to feel like she was "being gnawed on by a squirrel." She complained, "I am starting to really resent this, and I want to still have a happy relationship with my son, and if I want to stay happy, I need to stop this." When Margaret prepared for the arrival of a foster child who she planned to nurse and had "questionable HIV status," she weaned her three-year-old daughter. But because the daughter suffered from a dairy allergy, Margaret pumped and froze her milk to make "momsicles"—frozen breast milk treats—for her.

The negotiating is not always rainbows and sunshine. Family members also make moves to limit who gets to participate in the intimacy. Joanie, a Silicon Valley tech worker, is a divorced lesbian and mother of two. She and her partner instituted a strict and equitable division of labor: each woman carried one child (using her own egg and a known donor's sperm) and then breastfed that child. Joanie resented her partner's suggestion that they cofeed their second child. She took it as a selfish attempt by her partner to insert herself into Joanie's intimate nursing relationship. The two fought about it, and Joanie ended up being the only one to breastfeed her daughter.

The physical relationship of breastfeeding creates intimacy in a self-perpetuating, ongoing cycle. Intimacy influences physical and physiological responses—the milk flows along with emotional connection. This is not to say that the parent-child relationship is not physical when there is no breastfeeding. I did not breastfeed my first son. But I carried him in a wrap on my body most of the day for thirteen months, and he slept in my arms. Like breastfeeding, it took a physical toll on my body and our physiological selves—our heartbeats, scents, and skin-to-skin sensations—produced intimacy in a reciprocal way. The rocking, holding, feeding, diapering, and other bodily aspects of caring for children also make emotional connections. Mothering, as Barbara Katz Rothman says, is a physical endeavor—this is true whether or not we breastfeed.[31]

And some intimate collaborations are more parallel than entwined. Supportive dads, for instance, may pick up (but rarely procure) donor milk, provide the bulk of childcare for older children, wash the necessary bottles and tubes multiple times per day, and prepare meals that provide the breastfeeder with sufficient calories and nutrition. These third-party actions help bring the breastfeeding dyad closer together and can enhance family closeness.

Exceptional breastfeeders are experts on their own protocols and their own motivations. When any of us trespass social norms, we tend to know it and have our reasons. The same holds true for transgressive breastfeeders, who justify their practices by invoking certain common values such as intensive mothering, concerted cultivation, innovation, nutritionism, accomplishment, personal health, and self-reliance. When caregivers cannot breastfeed, they can still provide their children with breast milk. And those who are able to produce milk may offer it to others even if they cannot feed their own babies. In order to still provide "the best," caregivers will find ways to be successful. They tell me that flexibility and resilience are the secrets to successfully breastfeeding when things get complicated. Exercising these individual qualities becomes distinctly political in the face of institutional authority, the subject of the next chapter.

4 · MILKING THE SYSTEM

Expressing the Politics of Breastfeeding

If we could expand the boundaries that constrain the body's genius for breastfeeding, by loosening the grip of outdated conventions and attitudes, maybe we could allow it to drift in and out of all our lives, and revel with grace in its pleasures.

—Fiona Giles, *Fresh Milk: The Secret Life of Breasts*

Our society tries to suck all the joy out of breastfeeding. Infant feeding controversies create the illusion that there are black-and-white divides to debate with angst and conviction. The opposing options—breast or bottle, cover or no cover, pump or nurse on demand, baby-led weaning or developmental age–based weaning—preoccupy and distract, making a political and identity-staking minefield of what could be a more universally enjoyable experience. Exceptional breastfeeders will often try to abstain from participation in these controversies. Indeed, as Susan Falls suggests, perhaps it is better not to water down our sense of injustice by seeing "resistance everywhere."[1] Exceptional breastfeeders engage in practices like milk sharing, which "is powered by a politics of pragmatics, guided by a desire to meet specific goals."[2] Even if the political work is a side effect, daily actions and interpersonal struggles in pursuit of getting one's baby fed and cared for may add up to meaningful collective action.

EMBRACING ACTIVISM

"I despise capitalism. And I despise consumerism. I think health care is a right and not a privilege. I think that is why milk donation and extended nursing came so natural to me," said Stella, an accountant and mother of two. Though she explicitly connects her politics to breastfeeding in these statements, she did not initially approach breastfeeding as an opportunity to demonstrate her values. The "what is best for the child" philosophy drove her, and she did not yet see breastfeeding as activism. Later, she came to exemplify what I call an *embracer*—an exceptional breastfeeder who recognizes breastfeeding as a political exercise and as the impetus for political action, but only after breastfeeding becomes integral to her life.

Yesenia is also an embracer. She emphasized that she knew nothing about breastfeeding before she started. Her mother breastfed only for six weeks and stopped due to pain, so she was unable to advise Yesenia. After donating her milk and then becoming involved as an online administrator for Eats on Feets, Yesenia decided to pursue lactation consulting as a career. She went from "not knowing too much" to becoming quite skilled and knowledgeable over the course of breastfeeding her two children and donating her excess milk. She dreamed of becoming a lactation consultant who "isn't super pushy" but can lead others to see "what is possible." Until then, she continues working behind the scenes to connect those on the Eats on Feets message boards who want to share milk with those who need milk but are located in less populated areas and in geographically underrepresented areas.

This sort of awakening story was not at all unusual among the breastfeeders I interviewed. Sampling bias plays a role. Advocates exhibited some zeal in offering to participate in this study,[3] sometimes even initiating additional correspondence postinterview. They forwarded me photographs, interesting links, additional thoughts, and contact information for friends who might also wish to be interviewed. Breastfeeding in nonnormative ways takes a special effort. Exceptional breastfeeders may require additional social supports, for one thing. And conflicts with breastfeeders' intimate associates and with various authorities, such as hospital personnel and employers, often complicate matters. These breastfeeders are probably more likely to reflect on the meaning and purpose of their extraordinary efforts. They often want to articulate their reasons to others and to themselves.

Their desire to see policy changes increases as they become fully aware of the barriers to breastfeeding and as they experience intrusions on their private decisions. In a very obvious demonstration of politicization, this sort of experience may impact their voting. Several breastfeeders mentioned to me that, while conservative in other areas, they now lean progressive on "women's issues" or "reproductive rights."

Newfound awareness leads to other kinds of political action, some local and some global. Often, the work is about normalizing breastfeeding in all its varieties. Sabine traced her political consciousness to a terrible high-intervention hospital birth experience; breastfeeding became a successful redemption story. Eventually, she helped organize the well-publicized nurse-in at Facebook headquarters in 2012 to protest the social media giant's censorship of breastfeeding pics.

Stella acted more locally. After having gamely pumped her milk in a bathroom stall at work for her first child, she worked up the nerve to object to this arrangement with her second child. She and her coworkers retained a lawyer to convince the employer to provide a dedicated space. The final result? A supply closet given a coat of yellow paint.

Some political activism may seem fairly modest. Millicent, a Texas mother of three, never entertained the idea of breastfeeding before happening on a receptionist doing it. This transformative moment led Millicent to breastfeed at her own work desk "in case there is an opportunity to maybe accidentally help somebody else" by example. Exposure (literally, in this case) can effect cultural change by emboldening other breastfeeders to follow their lead.

ESPOUSING BREASTFEEDING POLITICS

Those who launch their breastfeeding journey from a preexisting political platform, I call *espousers*. Winnie, seventy-five at the time of the interview, described herself as an "original hippie." As a young mother, she surrounded herself with like-minded folks within enclaves in Hollywood, Chicago, Seattle, and Santa Cruz. Her comrades in natural motherhood resisted both medicalization and aspects of the feminist counterculture that denigrated motherhood as no better than servitude under patriarchy. "It was a more earthy group that was not too materialistic. I think we were kind of minimalists. Just had a spiritual look at raising children. I wouldn't say 'free,' but more of a communal attitude," Winnie recalled. The friends breast-fed each other's babies, joined the Women's Nursing Counsel—a cadre of in-home lactation support volunteers—and helped midwives and home birth doctors. She felt adamant about breastfeeding: "Why give into the marketing? It goes back to the viewpoint that we should encourage better things. We were born to improve the world."

Sometimes espousers' breastfeeding merges religious practice and political resistance. Conservative Christian evangelicals, Catholics, Mus-lims, Orthodox Jews, and Mormons I talked with spoke of breastfeeding as traditional and in accordance with their beliefs. Aaliyah consulted with her imam, who confirmed with Koranic scriptures that breastfeeding her four adopted children was morally correct. Breastfeeding spiritually bonded her to her children as their mother and bonded the children with one another, making them more related as "milk siblings" than they would otherwise be. As a Muslim, breastfeeding affirmed her piety. She further tapped into popular narratives of providing "the best" and emphasizing everything natural from cloth diapers to mother's milk (and nutrient-rich homemade formula made with hard-to-find ingredients). For Aaliyah, her performance of high-quality mothering amounted to more than concerted cultivation. She felt that by living a good life and by being a good mother, she proved that Islam strengthens families rather than threatens them.

Roxanne, a practicing Mormon who birthed four babies unassisted at home,[4] described an atmosphere of mothers feeding whichever babies passed nearby at church get-togethers, and her understanding of milk shar-ing extends that same philosophy. She noted, "Breastfeeding for me was a natural part of having a baby and . . . I always knew I would breastfeed. My mom did. All of my aunts did it. My grandma did. But I think it's also very much part of what's expected when you are in the home birth circles." Although Roxanne used the term *natural*, she immediately explained just how social her experience was. She described herself as a liberal femi-nist, and for her, breastfeeding evoked a women's realm: seemingly self-contained, existing in patriarchy but also apart from it, and protected from outside interference. Cofeeding, with its particular emphasis on sharing, was a way to live traditionally and religiously in this insular feminine milieu. Roxanne pointed out that breastfeeding conforms to the social expectations of "home birth circles," a further instance of a circumscribed boundary around women doing their thing in their own way, leaving the man-made world of hospitals and doctors out of procreative matters altogether.

Members of intentional communities centered on birth and breast-feeding declare outright that breastfeeding is a political matter. Tiana, a breastfeeding mother of two living in Atlanta, described a collective of "black moms who are living and parenting outside the mainstream." In this context, she expected to breastfeed well beyond the broader norm of one year. The group members gather to talk about their "goddess" work as spiritual mothers revitalizing an unadulterated African legacy. Journal-ist and breastfeeding advocate Kimberly Seals Allers, writing for *Ebony Magazine*, told of an encounter with a black woman who asked her to stop talking about "that slavery shit," referring to breastfeeding. Breastfeeding seemed like going backward to a time when black women were forced to be wet nurses for enslavers' children. Allers goes on to decry the "stunted and complex mothering experience" suffered by generations of black women.[5] Ditching this baggage, Allers suggests, will help turn around the compara-tively abysmal black infant mortality statistics. She is careful not to blame mothers but instead to place the burden of responsibility on American institutions that continue to damage black motherhood with their unrelent-ing, enmeshed systems of oppression.[6]

Black women seek to overcome the historical anguish of motherhood, birth, and breastfeeding in slavery and Jim Crow. Saidiya Hartman writes about the "afterlife of slavery," in which the violent effects of the institution continue to resonate in everyday experiences in the contemporary world.[7] As part of recovery from these abuses, Tiana's community works not only to normalize breastfeeding but to exalt it. In a ritual performance of regal motherhood—epitomized by pregnant Beyoncé's 2017 Grammy appear-ance dressed as a queen or goddess—some members of this broader com-munity document their pregnancy and breastfeeding journeys with lush professional photo shoots of themselves adorned in African-inspired fin-ery, with natural hairstyles or head wraps, painted pregnant bellies, and intimate soft-focus portraits with their nursing infants (and toddlers). The production of this visual culture provides self-validation. At the same time, when shared publicly, it strengthens this community of black mothers and promotes a "natural" and ethnic motherhood that includes breastfeeding. Examples can be seen in posts on the social media sites of Black Women Do Breastfeed (BWDBF) and the website A Mother's Peace, among others.

Most of the comments affirm the "beauty" of motherhood and breastfeeding. They actively decolonize their motherhood by turning toward the natural and throwing off biomedicine and commercial products like formula. In mining the legacy of collective support and traditional knowledge and wisdom, they espouse a return to a self-sustaining black maternal world.

Facebook groups like BWDBF (168,000 followers) and the Badass Breastfeeder (more than 257,000 likes) foster an unapologetic espouser mind-set. "No excuse ladies! Get those babies breastfed," reads an October 25, 2016, post on the page for a real-life, dues-paying group calling itself the Breastfeeding MAFIA (Mothers Against Feeding Infants Artificially). The post includes a link to a picture and post from BWDBF that highlights a breastfeeding mother of four and full-time student who also works full time; the photograph is of a black woman in her twenties, baby to breast, sitting on a sofa with a laptop in front of her on a coffee table and a textbook in hand. The MAFIA's "Breast Practices and Standards of Excellence," published on the Facebook page, includes rules about meeting attendance and confidentiality—and jocular item Number 11: "BREASTFEED OR DIE!"

Critics of "lactivism" often convey annoyance with such language, which they see as shaming bottle-feeders, as if one practice cannot be celebrated without putting down another.[8] This worry about undue pressure, however, rarely reflects an intersectional analysis: most members of the Breastfeeding MAFIA are women of color. Their advocacy around breastfeeding is not rooted in privilege but seeks to redress centuries of procreative oppression.

Now for a wildly different standpoint: Kerry, twenty-three, a white, evangelical Tea Party proponent and nursing mother of two who lives in rural Texas, wore hunting gear during our conversation. She believes that women should be at home with their children and that the government should stay out of our lives. She homeschools her kids. Her church and Bible study group are a big part of her life. Breastfeeding started out as a way to "provide immunities" in place of vaccination, and it was congruent with her homesteading sensibilities.

Procreative politics have a way of making strange bedfellows: Kerry considers herself a "crunchy" mom. This 1990s slang once alluded to granola munching lefties but now is an umbrella adjective that describes just about anything that is "natural" and a bit outside the commercial mainstream (or cleverly co-opted and branded as natural by the commercial mainstream).

Examples include acupuncture and veganism. Kerry belongs to a local community group of extended breastfeeders who engage in multiple crunchy practices. They use cloth diapers, cosleep, and wear their babies in wraps. She said, "They try to eat healthy and try to make their own baby food instead of using preservatives, and you learn—try to learn—so much about better ways to live." For religious conservatives like Kerry, these "better ways to live" stem from a desire for independence from the godless state. Some of her comrades in baby wraps, though, are progressive environmentalists and lefty antivaxxers. She has borrowed components from progressive ideologies and used them to her own political ends. For her, it was not about resisting capitalism but about a way to recapture a more traditional way of life. For Kerry, traditional is maintaining a patriarchal white Christianity.

Other espousers come to breastfeeding from a conservative background but reconfigure its politics in the opposite direction. Devin explained, "The church that I grew up in is a very conservative church, but growing up in the seventies, women were breastfeeding in church. That was the thing. It was very DIY. It was Mormons. It was the pioneer spirit to feed your own baby from your own breast." Devin and their wife keep backyard chickens and can their homegrown produce. They are "very DIY" but with progressive objectives that reject capitalism and raise environmental consciousness. For espousers like Devin, their breastfeeding is green, it is self-sufficient, it resists corporate marketing, and it is potentially outside of patriarchal control.

"ANTIACTIVISM, YOU KNOW?": INTRINSICALLY POLITICAL BREASTFEEDING

All infant feeding practices in the contemporary West are political, whether or not the caregiver recognizes this fact. It is like the apocryphal Niels Bohr story about a lucky horseshoe, in which he said, "I am told it works even if you don't believe in it." Public debates make it so that even the old standby of formula and bottles—the unquestioned norm for decades—now signifies a stance, however unwittingly. I use the shorthand *intrinsics* for breastfeeders who experience their exceptional practices as incidental to their political awareness (anthropologist Susan Falls calls this sort of political work "microactivism," an apt descriptor of this highly localized flavor of resistance).[9]

Cricket even intimated that politics and extended breastfeeding can be antithetical. "Just because I breastfed for four years even doesn't mean I consider myself a lactivist," she insisted. She shied away from a local protest against the firing of a popular lactation consultant when it turned into a rally in support of breastfeeding:

> I was there for a while and I realized everyone was making an issue—there were a lot of these signs saying "breast is best" and "babies need milk." It was never about that. I just went because I wanted to support someone who had been very helpful in my journey. . . . I didn't go to say, "[The hospital] needs to let babies have breast milk." They are hiring a replacement for [the fired lactation consultant]. It's not like they are giving up breastfeeding. I was kind of turned off by it all. I had decided that was not my scene. I went there to support [the lactation consultant]. I didn't go to stand and have people honk their horns at me because I'm into breastfeeding. And because I think I am superior because I was breastfeeding. . . . I was formula fed and I'm fine, which means that I am fine with anybody who chooses to formula feed. But I think the implication sometimes is that if I did it for so long that I am somehow making some kind of political statement. Or there is some activism about it. It just wasn't. It was easy. It was the path of least resistance for me. Antiactivism, you know?

Cricket did not want to be seen as an activist because it would imply a superiority complex when her extended breastfeeding (and milk donation) were not part of some intentional trailblazing. Rather, she was always following "the path of least resistance," a passive, natural meandering full of common sense, not an active, political, and statement-making march forward. She reserved the term *activism* for the deserving who are setting out to make a difference and, somewhat mockingly, for the silly or bored bandwagon-jumpers she observed turning the rally sideways (the oft-pejorative "lactivism"). In this schema, those at the rally thought that they were activists instead of overprivileged women with too much time on their hands. (I attended this rally and interviewed some of these protestors on the spot. I got the sense that they felt like the hospital was undermining breastfeeding in the community by firing this favorite, very talented lactation consultant.)

Irrespective of their intention, exceptional breastfeeding interrupts the status quo. A young married lesbian couple, Aurora and Beth Ann, both twenty-five, decided to share in the breastfeeding of their daughter. They already considered themselves to be radical homebodies for settling down and starting a family so young; Aurora said, "We are just old people inside." But they never expected what would happen when their friend, a birth photographer, posted pictures of them each breastfeeding on her business's website: media outlets began calling. The story went viral, and reporters from a few different newspapers and popular websites interviewed them. One reporter decided to spin the story into a debate questioning the wisdom of "taking drugs" (the mostly innocuous domperidone) to induce lactation. The comments sections went wild. The couple originally kept their plans to breastfeed quiet even from their families, but, ironically, their breastfeeding sparked the most public of debates. I was impressed with their self-described millennial approach to these internet conversations; they took criticisms and praise mostly in stride, focusing their energy on their newborn. Arguably, they were shaking things up just by living their lives.

Indeed, breastfeeders may passively accept politicization of their breastfeeding by other people, even if the breastfeeder declines to engage politically. Jessica voted "all over the place" and prided herself in having moderate views on everything; she supported breastfeeding but was no "activist." She commented, "I don't nurse in public to make a scene, but when it makes its own statement, it's kind of nice."

Some aspects of exceptional breastfeeding may be easier to openly advocate than others. Liza induced lactation and used a supplemental nursing system (SNS) to nurse her adoptive son, who arrived from Korea at the age of seven months. She did so because she thought even nonnutritive suckling puts parents "more in tune with the child's needs than bottle-feeding." Her midwife kept a photograph of Liza and her baby posted prominently in her office as "incentive for anyone having difficulty." Wary of social repercussions, however, Liza was not quick to divulge that she was still breastfeeding her son even though he was now seven years old. She quietly promoted breastfeeding, providing emotional support to breastfeeders she knew and writing a letter to a government agency to encourage research into milk sharing. Though she embraced breastfeeding politics in some ways, her most boundary-pushing breastfeeding practice—extended "comfort nursing"—got into territory that felt less safe to publicize.

All exceptional breastfeeders—who seem to be a sizeable portion of the breastfeeding population[10]—are doing political work. They normalize breastfeeding whether the activism is intentional or incidental. But this normalization happens in fits and starts, with new boundaries and rules emerging all the time. For example, more people accept nursing in public and more laws protect the unfettered right to do so. Breastfeeding in public is now legally protected in forty-nine U.S. states (only Idaho has yet to provide an exclusion to public nudity prohibitions). Yet as public awareness of milk sharing grows, so too does the pushback from public health advocates who feel highly uncomfortable with this free market—"free," as in no cost *and* unregulated—of "body fluids." These same institutional forces boast some successes in controlling semen, another "dangerous" body fluid, especially when it comes to women's use of it; some states prohibit at-home inseminations or require unenforceable legal and medical "permission." Staving off regulation that limits breastfeeding might prove to be the most pressing political concern for advocates.

POWER PLAYS

"You are talking to the moms of this baby!" Amelia and Sami insisted with anger at their "thoughtless" medical providers. Exceptional breastfeeders' politics get played out in their interactions with authorities—for example, employers, medical personnel, midwives and lactation consultants, social workers, clerics, and parenting experts. Some of these power struggles between breastfeeders and institutions (and the representatives of those institutions) threaten the parents' identity and their ability to care for their children as they see fit.

Same-sex couples and transgender parents often have to fight for recognition in their chosen roles. Sami, a transgender breastfeeding mother and genetic parent, recalled:

> Half the fucking time, we are seeing a doctor for some reason and they will say some shit like, "Who is the daddy?" Or like, we were asking something about [our son's] height, and they would say something like, "Is his *daddy* tall?" And we would be like, "There is no fucking daddy. You are talking to the moms of

this baby! We just told you. We introduced ourselves as, 'We are his moms.' And you are talking to both of us about his medical care, and you are going to ask about fucking daddy?!" It is insanely offensive. It is thoughtless.

Sami and her wife, Amelia, took the time to preemptively explain their atypical family-building process partly to avoid any mutual embarrassment during their doctor visits. Though medical personnel appeared to understand, they still failed to be respectful. Some providers reverted to tried-and-true scripts—in this case joking, casual references to "daddy"—without considering their patients' individual situations. Each of these small indignities adds up to a whole that destroys the quality of care.

Sami and Amelia blamed this pattern on institutional policy rather than on a host of bad actors. The training of personnel at their local medical center, they noted, was inconsistent. Kaiser Permanente hospitals in California, by contrast, where Amelia received pregnancy medical care prior to moving outside of the state, did a much better job. Everyone from the receptionist to the doctors knew how to properly address them and refrained from asking nosy questions. Los Angeles–based lesbian cofeeding couple Jeri (the egg-providing mother) and Allie (the gestational, birthing mother) also praised Kaiser's stick-to-the-pertinent-facts policies. In this scenario, regulation expands breastfeeders' autonomy rather than limiting it by trying to force everyone into old-fashioned roles.

All four of these white, middle-class mothers exuded self-confidence and shared the expectation that the medical personnel who *work for them* should treat them with the same courtesy extended to patients who conform to gender norms. Exceptional breastfeeders with less social capital cannot count on a consumerist identity, even less so when they must interface with public assistance providers. For example, a working-class couple, both of whom are transgender, sought peer guidance online, asking if anyone knew the Women, Infants, and Children Food and Nutrition Service (WIC) policy on transgender support. The gestational parent transitioned to male and the sperm-providing parent transitioned to female, and the fear was that the workers at their county WIC office in their newly adopted Southern home state[11] would treat them poorly. In their case, an institutional policy toward equitable treatment was crucial. They could neither count on individual goodwill nor wield class privilege; they relied on the providers for their care, and these same providers could potentially deny or delay services via loopholes, red tape, and just plain meanness. (They ended up calling ahead of time to explain their circumstances; when the couple arrived, everyone treated them well.)

As anthropologist Charlotte Faircloth establishes in her ethnographic studies of British and French attachment and mothers' breastfeeding, much of breastfeeding in the West these days is identity work.[12] This identity work, as we have seen, varies across intersections of class status, racial histories, gender, sexuality, religion, and geography. The breastfeeding practices of a young, white, rural, Texan evangelical or of a cosmopolitan, city-dwelling, radical black activist confirm their identities in vastly disparate ways because they have to contend with differing systems of oppression. What sorts of breastfeeding their respective communities consider to be "normal" also varies.

Normalizing breastfeeding in general and, more to the point, normalizing exceptional breastfeeding—modifying how it is done or redefining what breastfeeding is—cannot be exclusively a grassroots hearts-and-minds effort. To be sure, seeing someone else nursing a toddler, learning of a butch lesbian breastfeeding, or scrolling through scores of online images of black women tandem nursing opens up these options to many caregivers who had not dared to plan for these possibilities. But when breastfeeders decide to go public with milk sharing or cofeeding or any other unapproved practice, they risk real sanctions that range in severity depending on the breastfeeders' social standing.

The significant gaps between institutional and societal goals versus individual goals regarding breastfeeding create ironic circumstances. One obvious example is the deliberate obfuscation of the "cost" of breastfeeding. Is breastfeeding the *free* option when every choice relies on unpaid labor and loss of income or productivity?[13] It requires the breastfeeder to be at home with the baby and nurse on demand or else pump at work during no-break "breaks" and stay up all night nursing a reverse-cycling infant. The costs are high in either case. Society now generally glorifies exclusive breastfeeding. "I am so proud of the fact that we have never used a single drop of formula in this house ever," said Valerie. But as a society, we do not make breastfeeding easier to do in public. There is more worry about breast exposure when it is for nursing than when it is for selling beer (or burgers, cars, power tools, and music albums).

These kinds of difficult-to-resolve dilemmas feed into the politicization of boundary-pushing breastfeeders in particular. Strategies for dealing with these conflicts may be indirect—sidestepping authority or quiet coping—or they may involve more head-on efforts like managing authority or asserting authority. Some even become experts or immerse themselves into countermovements. Breastfeeders may select from any combination of these options depending on the vagaries of their particular situations. One breastfeeder might have a different strategy with each child because their infants' needs vary and because their lives change.

SIDESTEPPING AUTHORITY

"Liability, blah, blah, blah," intoned Jeri. She and her wife, Allie, found it irritating that a hospital treated breast milk like medicine instead of like food, an orientation seen in the medical literature.[14] They wanted to donate their extra milk to a lesbian couple's infant twins—the new parents, who planned to cofeed, were having a hard time producing enough right away. But the hospital representatives invoked strict written policies in order to override the pediatrician's OK. The two erstwhile donors responded by conspiring with friendly hospital staff to sneak the milk into the neonatal intensive care unit (NICU). Jeri and Allie were driven to support their friends' breastfeeding, and they were not very swayed by what they saw as preposterous misgivings over the safety of the milk. This was milk that they provided to their own baby after all. Institutions like the hospital in this example hold to standards and policies that conflict with what parents want for their children. (This same hospital, however, has the policies mentioned earlier that limit gender stereotyping.) The parents sidestepped authority to get their way while also avoiding material repercussions and reducing direct conflict. Like Rayna Rapp's "moral pioneers" who resist prenatal testing,[15] they did not accept medical risk narratives without question. They refused total medical management of their maternal bodies. Plus the overwrought, liability-avoiding policies did not seem to them to be based in sound medical science.

These Mothers Will Make Their Own Informed
Decisions about What Is Risky, Thank You[16]

There is a trade-off in subverting institutional surveillance: lying or leaving out information may make it difficult to access the services one needs. My son's birth mother relinquished him (a consistent pattern for her; my boys have at least eight other biological siblings adopted by other families), but she disappeared before signing all the appropriate documents. It was logical for me to assume that I would be adopting him. I reasoned that if I asked the court for permission to breastfeed, they might deny the request, and then I would be subject to closer monitoring by social workers. On the other hand, if I followed the maxim, "It is easier to ask forgiveness than ask permission," perhaps I could continue breastfeeding. I made the latter choice. But then I ended up having to lie to his county-provided occupational therapist even though she could have helped me improve his latch. I also had to rush around to hide the pumping equipment and then feed him with bottles when social workers dropped by my house to check on us.

Margaret chose to be honest about breastfeeding her foster child. And for her trouble, the social workers removed the baby from her home. It is a prickly subject from the get-go. Sheena asked the social workers who were hosting a foster care information night if breastfeeding "is something the foster parents could do." She said, "They just looked at us like we had sprouted another head." Sheena's wife, Romy, added, "They held it against us forever." They learned early on not to ask.

Deep involvement with the system helps some breastfeeders navigate the pitfalls that might threaten their breastfeeding autonomy. At first, Lanie had the same experience as Sheena and Romy at an adoption information night: "We went up and we shared that we wanted to adopt an infant because I wanted to breastfeed, and the woman looked at me and said, 'That is just sick!... You would nurse somebody else's baby? You didn't give birth to that child. This is not your child. This is not your child until they are adopted. That takes a lot of years and blah, blah, blah, and absolutely not. You cannot nurse a foster child.' ... We walked out of there, and I was crying."

I was not surprised to hear of the disgusted reaction from the woman running this informational meeting. I too asked about foster breastfeeding during preplacement training sessions. Though the social workers only gave me strange looks and avoided answering me (versus going on and on about it being "sick"), I got the message.[17] Hurt and confused, Lanie called up a friend who she remembered had breastfed her foster children. It turned out that the woman and her family members knew to lie to the social workers. Lanie was not willing to take this tack.

Knowing what information to share, and with whom, can smooth the way to exceptional breastfeeding and other offbeat parenting practices. Comothers Kris and Rachel dealt with many twists and turns during their family building. A birth mother scammed them by pretending to choose them as adoptive parents, Rachel experienced a stillbirth, and social services reunified one of their foster sons with his birth family. (Kris and Rachel thought they were going to adopt him.) In a trial-by-fire kind of way, they uncovered the intricacies of policies said and unsaid, written and unwritten. Later, they made sure to appear to be adhering to them all. Any divergence from these standards, they kept prudently secret. By staying covert, they could breastfeed their foster children with impunity.

Ignoring Authority

My eight-year-old son Leo knows all about appearing to listen—make eye contact and nod—but then choosing to dismiss instructions. It works better at school, where there are many kids in his class, than it does at home, where he gets called to account. Ignoring authoritative advice and authoritative institutions as a sidestepping maneuver is particularly effective in this anomic society. Nobody cares to keep track.

Alice, who ordinarily never shies away from a fight, sidestepped authority to protect her daughter. Alice explained to her puzzled husband that the reason she declined to inform hospital staff that she was breastfeeding her daughter's baby in the hospital had nothing to do with shame or doubts about whether she would win that battle with nurses and doctors. "I knew I was healthy and fine because I was nursing also my [infant] daughter. I just didn't want the judgment placed on my [postpartum] daughter, and I didn't want to make them make her feel like she wasn't going to be able to do it and maybe discourage her. So I just chose not to tell them anything," she said. Leaving the authorities out of the loop prevented them from disrupting her daughter's potential.

For Ariel, sidestepping amounted to selecting privacy and avoiding the middleman. She chose informal milk sharing even though she lived close to the regional milk bank because it allowed her to skip the administrative screening process. She preferred to collaborate directly with other mothers because it felt less intrusive.

Kadijah concertedly avoided books about childbirth and breastfeeding in an effort to reject society's efforts at "public education": "[Not research-ing] would allow me to be very primal and just be open and kind of let my body experience the process. So I just kind of carry that over into my moth-ering. Instinctively, I am a mammal; it's not like any of the other mammals get some sort of training. That they read books, go to classes. . . . I think it was a good call for me." She wanted to have what she saw as more "instinc-tive" reactions in the moment without intellectualizing the process.

Ruha Benjamin identifies a resistance practice of "informed refusal," in which people of color actively choose not to participate in scientific stud-ies that have a history of learning from their bodies but then not benefiting people of color.[18] For similar reasons, Kadijah refused scientific informa-tion. She sought advice on particular questions about breastfeeding but only from her wise "mommy friends." In this way, she limited her complicity in self-surveillance even as she took an essentialist view of herself as a mam-mal. The philosopher Michel Foucault writes that "we are agents of our own normalization"; in our bid to control our "unruly bodies," we serve the insti-tutions that seek to constrain us.[19] He calls this site of struggle "biopower." Kadijah, and others who opt out of researching all aspects of breastfeeding or who dismiss advice that would regulate their bodies, carved out a breast-feeding existence that takes back some of that power. Kadijah welcomed unruliness, as she chose to become "primal," a way of trusting her body over medicine and how-to guides that homogenize the birth and breastfeeding experiences. It is important to remember that the aim of her essentializing language was to take control back from constraining institutions, not to cast herself as helpless to her biology. Some in the black community dis-dain breastfeeding for its historical relation to closer-to-nature narratives and overlapping oppressions of black people, poor people, and women. The wider black community for a long time preferred the sanitized distance that bottle-feeding appears to enable. Kadijah and others I interviewed recalled their elders talking about binding their breasts to stop the milk. She rejected this practice and instead reclaimed her body's wisdom—not reducing her-self to a mammal so much as strategically deploying her body's functions.

Preemptive Moves

Exceptional breastfeeders may not want to have to defend their practices. In this way of thinking, what they choose to do is none of the medical service providers' business. When Joanie's newborn needed to stay in the hospital for a few days due to jaundice, Joanie preempted hospital intervention in her infant-feeding goals: "My milk took a while to come in, and I really didn't want to do the formula debate. I didn't want her to have formula when she was so tiny. So I had a friend who was breastfeeding her son—he was, I think, six months old at the time. She smuggled in some breast milk for us."

Joanie, her partner, and their friends went to some trouble merely to avoid her having to ask the hospital not to give formula to her baby. The risk of asking was that the hospital workers may have refused or argued coercively. Some birth centers and hospitals can be slow to discharge jaundiced newborns (a very common diagnosis that is usually mild but can be life-threatening). It can be a problem before milk comes in or, in some cases, when a quality of the milk contributes to the buildup of bilirubin. The liver cannot efficiently metabolize excess bilirubin, which can cause brain damage in extreme cases. Medical providers' concerns about jaundice contribute to formula-pushing, which, in turn, threatens breastfeeding goals.[20]

Public and private medical service providers increasingly over the past few decades cast infant feeding as a public health matter rather than a private choice. This viewpoint emboldens them to interfere. Kylie's job could be on the line, or at least the respect she received at work would be at risk, if she were to divulge her use of raw cows' milk (thought by some to be healthier than commercially available homogenized milk) to supplement her breast milk. With the support of her pediatrician, she combined it with the Weston A. Price Foundation's infant formula mix.[21] This controversial organization promotes "perfect" nutrition in general and touts its formula as conforming to this perfection. It bases its formulations on indigenous diets. Kylie worked at a NICU with some colleagues who she saw as too conservative and unforgiving: "I feel like raw milk might have been a little bit too much for them. My lactation consultants that I worked with at work knew that I was giving her raw milk formula, and one of my close friends that works with me in the NICU knew. I just didn't make an announcement. I actually tried to avoid it with most people who were asking me."

She continued to pump at work, so everyone assumed she only fed her baby breast milk. Nobody was keeping close tabs on her as long as she seemed to be complying with expectations.

Raw, or unpasteurized, milk is heavily regulated in her community—she had to buy it as "pet milk" at health food stores in small quantities with the help of friends and family who made some of the purchases. Kylie, like some others engaging in rule-bending breastfeeding, recruited supporters who provided a practical and emotional buffer between her and the enforcers of restrictive policies.

Replacing Authority

Breastfeeders engaging in nonnormative practices can also avoid negative judgment and institutional control by seeking out alternative health providers, switching doctors, attending a different church, signing on with a better adoption agency, or changing jobs. Jessica, a nurse, had to make her way across a large hospital building to the designated pumping room during her fifteen-hour shifts: "As an ER nurse, you would think that the job is really stressful, but the most stressful part of my entire job was pumping. Like, making sure I had the time . . . and having a hard time getting enough [milk] out because of stress." Her colleagues were unkind about her forty-five-minute breaks. The stress of this setup led her to change departments by the time her next child was born; she found a more sympathetic boss, more frequent break times, and nicer coworkers. For these reasons, she "didn't even care" that she had to pump in a bathroom or that the work was less satisfying.

Conventional medical providers like pediatricians, obstetricians, and nurses typically lack enough experience and training to provide truly supportive breastfeeding care.[22] They have other demands on them, and the time-consuming, emotional work of troubleshooting breastfeeding difficulties often falls outside their purview. As such, their advice, though bearing the weight of authority, can cause more harm than good. Exceptional breastfeeders learn to avoid them and their iffy opinions.

Doulas and the specifically trained lactation consultants have taken on more of this work—for those who can afford additional members of their care team, since insurance coverage is spotty. These advocates come with their own "contradictory maternalist and medicalized discourses"[23] and values, of course, with which breastfeeders still have to contend. Always, there is a precarious balance between support and surveillance. Multiple respondents expressed discomfort with their lactation consultant's snap judgments and with the invasions of personal space. At what point do gestures intended to be supportive become oppressive? For example, some exclusive pumpers feel antagonized by the constant "encouragement" to reintroduce the baby to the breast. Many potential supporters assume that the physical connection is better, but some of these would-be breastfeeders cannot bear the sensation or like Ariel, prefer the routine they have established.

Yet there are plenty of exceptional breastfeeders who credit their lactation consultants or lay experts like La Leche League (LLL) leaders with helping them surmount the obstacles in the way of breastfeeding. Joanie's enthusiasm was not unusual: "Oh, lifesavers! Lifesavers. Just the whole, 'Cram them on your boob, and let's eat.' [Infants] are so fragile, I was just afraid I was going to kill them constantly on accident. Just squishing them, being too rough with them. But [the lactation consultants] are all just, 'No, just slap them on your boob.' Invaluable lactation consultants. Just to be like, 'This is normal. Here are some pro tips, but everything you are going through is totally normal.' That was priceless."

These heroines offer "pro tips" instead of stringent guidelines. They place most of the credit with the breastfeeder. More than anything, breastfeeders need reassurance that things are progressing "normally." It is not unusual for Americans to embark on parenthood having zero experience with infants and infant care. One woman in a lactation support group showed her breastfed daughter's poopy diaper to each arriving mother, asking, "Does this look normal to you?" Being able to identify problematic symptoms is, well, a problem.

One lactation consultant I observed leading classes always focused on validating the breastfeeders' "journeys," whether they were establishing a freezer stash for their return to their paid jobs, trying to induce lactation, nursing on demand, or making sure their baby received enough formula to supplement low breast milk supply. She expended little energy advising them about *how* they should be breastfeeding.

Consultations do not always go well, however. Lactation consultants' hospital-style efficiency can be at odds with the patients' need for nurturing. At the same time that lactation consultants work to demedicalize breastfeeding, they work deep within a medicalized system.[24] For Mona, initiating breastfeeding in a clinical setting "was just a failed affair." Although she said that she was "not too impressed" with the lactation consultant, most of the blame lay with the system's controlled chaos. Too many nurses, doctors, phlebotomists, and others interrupted her rest and, worse, provided conflicting advice. The lactation consultant brusquely and, according to Mona, unhelpfully told her to keep trying. Nurses who visited a few minutes later pushed formula.

Some breastfeeders find themselves needing to sidestep LLL *doctrine* (more so than the leaders themselves). Each of the thousands of chapters runs independently—often, I suspect, in accordance with local cultural norms. Christine Bobel, a sociologist who writes about the "paradoxes" of so-called natural motherhood, questions LLL's emphasis on empowering breastfeeders to reject conventional medicine (which approves of formula) while disempowering those who have to mix-feed or return to paid jobs.[25] LLL offers a path for members to become peer "leaders"; prospects undergo a special application process and training regimen. They become enculturated into certain standards, but these standards may restrict adaptive breastfeeding. Susan struggled with this contradiction. She took her position as a La Leche leader seriously, staying clear of the rumor mill by declining an opportunity to nurse a friend's baby: "I would not want to give the wrong impression about—having that reflect on me as a leader—because we, I don't want to use the word 'professional' because we are not professionals—we are mother support, but there is just this standard of wanting to be accessible to everybody. I wouldn't want [someone to say], 'You can go to La Leche League, but the leaders are kind of crazy because they will just nurse your baby.'"

Susan only wanted to give her milk to mothers who had made every conceivable attempt to bring in a sufficient milk supply. She donated her milk selectively, again to avoid running afoul of LLL values: "I don't want to make it so easy for her that she resorts to [donated milk] quicker than she might otherwise and have it be hurting her own supply, because if I do that, then I am really no different than a formula company."

Spring, a mother of one from Florida, deliberately separated her role "as a mother" from her role as an LLL leader. This meant that she could not talk about her experience with pumping because it was not part of the LLL party line. She said it was important that LLL leaders avoid "setting themselves apart" as role models. LLL generally disdains pumping as alienating mother from baby and instead strongly encourages on-demand breastfeeding.

The group also warns that using supplements diminishes milk supply and thus the breastfeeding relationship. Spring could not be forthright about her own breastfeeding in LLL circles because she gave her baby almond milk formula. Though she and Susan each made their own forays over the breastfeeding boundaries set by the authority of LLL, they did so only with great care.

Amy has insufficient glandular tissue (IGT), and after some poor interactions early on, she sidestepped LLL. Their inflexibility and inexperience frustrated her: "Some of them don't have any experience with it. It's a mentality of, 'Well. You nurse more. If you have the demand, then you will have the supply.' The end." Doctors and lactation consultants alike negated her reality. She finally obtained a measure of vindication when a support group for breastfeeders with IGT formed on the internet and some clinical research on the condition was published. In the meantime, however, Amy learned not to solicit advice from self-professed experts who knew too little.

Lactation professionals constitute another authority that some exceptional breastfeeders choose to bypass. This is especially the case if they cannot offer culturally competent services. Efforts to decolonize this profession include organizing conferences and online groups and offering training specifically for people of color who wish to become IBCLCs (International Board Certified Lactation Consultants) or experts who are not formally certified (Acquanda Stanford, an activist, anthropologist, and doula, offers web-based classes).[26] Trevor MacDonald, a transgender chestfeeding dad, publicly lobbied his local LLL chapter to accept him as a peer leader and, in 2014, to change their gender discriminatory policy. Since then, he has been at the vanguard championing trans and queer breastfeeding and chestfeeding.[27] Change is afoot. Perhaps lactation consultants lead the charge because many of them were themselves exceptional breastfeeders.

Sidestepping authority, in all its permutations, allows exceptional breastfeeders to stay on their unique paths without undue interference. While they remain hyperaware that they are breaching protocols, exceptional breastfeeders draw from other convincing moral imperatives like concerted cultivation, bodily independence, parenting autonomy, and the "breast is best" axiom to justify their rebelliousness.

QUIET COPING

Exceptional breastfeeders get tired of surveillance and intervention by medical and legal institutions that formalize and enforce the norms. Breast-feeders address disagreements with doctors and other authorities (like social workers) either by making concessions or with reluctant acceptance. Anthropologists Cecilia Tomori, Aunchalee Palmquist, and Sally Dowling pooled their ethnographic research findings to explore some of the "moral landscapes" of breastfeeding stigma.[28] In looking at the practices of breast milk sharing, nighttime breastfeeding, and long-term breastfeeding in the United States and the United Kingdom, they found that breastfeeders will avoid health professionals or keep their practices secret in order to mitigate the stigma.[29] The exceptional breastfeeders I interviewed did not want to be judged either. They employ a wide range of avoidance and limited appease-ment strategies, all types of quiet coping.

Agree to Disagree

"The doctor is mystified because she feels like [breastfeeding] doesn't pro-vide any nutrition anymore," said Kendra, a professor and divorced mother of two who nursed her toddler. Instead of resorting to deception or arguing with the doctor, Kendra thought to herself that the doctor was just not "get-ting it." She told me, "Breastfeeding can be symbolic; it's just a loving expres-sion; it helps her calm her down. It's more about the love and the closeness." Love and closeness and symbolism are rather hard to measure in medical or scientific terms. The pediatrician shrugged at Kendra's extended breastfeed-ing with all these intangible reasons for it; Kendra shrugged right back at the doctor's narrow-minded ignorance. It is a well-worn fact that conven-tional biomedical practice tends toward that which is evidence-based, sci-entifically tested, and encoded into policy. It did not surprise Kendra that the doctor lacked a holistic approach. She knew the doctor did hold with symbolism. But a shrug instead of condemnation may be progress. And this tolerance is probably more readily available to breastfeeders with the right social privileges.

Biding Time

At times, negative or judgmental interactions elicit much more than non-committal shrugs. Emotions become heightened for the parents when the situation gets serious, such as when the infant or parent is sick or when a foster placement becomes insecure. The professionals' legal liability increases at the same time, possibly driving a wedge between their interests and the goals of the parents. Social workers in charge of foster care arrangements may be probreastfeeding but may worry about the birth parents' reactions or a judge's disapproval. Vanessa abided by the social worker's request that she wait until the birth parents' parental rights were legally terminated before commencing the nursing relationship with her adoptive daughter-to-be.

Resignation

Breastfeeding versus formula conflicts occasionally involve serious health matters. Often, the struggle signifies retention or loss of power over one's body and over parenting autonomy. Relative privilege and social location usually factor in. Kendra, who has plenty of social capital herself, coped with the doctor's naysaying by dismissing its relevance to her own experience. But Lily became depressed about the formula recommendations every time she visited the doctor's office. As a single mother and person of color, disapproval from authorities stung more than it might for a woman whose fitness for motherhood was never questioned. It was not like Kendra's situation, where she could dismiss the doctor and the doctor, for her part, remained uninterested in intervening. Instead, for Lily, authorities' unfair assumptions about her motherhood loomed in the background. Although she kept breastfeeding, Lily second-guessed her decision and sometimes felt lost and alone as a result.[30] She tried to focus more on self-care, which was not easy when she had to put in overtime to make ends meet. Just because someone is quietly coping does not mean they feel unharmed. Sometimes they are keeping their heads down merely to avoid further trouble. Lily endured others' judgment because she had little social capital and little recourse.

Avoidance

Katie, a rural Texan and Far Right conservative, distrusts doctors and their motives. She learned to avoid frustrating encounters long before she was ready to breastfeed. "Diabetic babies *die*," came the ominous warning from her obstetrician, who was concerned about Katie's Type I diabetes. The doctor continued, "I just had a girl next door, and she lost her baby at thirty-nine weeks." Katie said, "I just walked around full of anxiety, afraid the baby was going to die every day because he led [me] to believe that way. . . . There were just tests after tests just to make sure he was alive, and I couldn't handle all of that again, so I switched." She got a new doctor who toned it down a bit. The high-risk label, which she got slapped with as a diabetic, empowers providers to intervene more thoroughly in pregnancies and births,[31] and this oft-patronizing pattern extends, postpartum, to breastfeeding. After having been pushed around during the pregnancy and birth, she resisted getting breastfeeding advice from clinical providers. She missed appointments, educated herself from internet sources, and followed her intuition. Katie's immediate response to her doctors' opinions was to say nothing and then do what she wanted to.

Limited Concessions

Others offer minimal compliance. Jen, for instance, who gritted her teeth as she remembered, "The doctor really wanted me to give formula" (in order to more quickly treat jaundice in her newborn), did so in the hospital with reluctance and resentment. She suspected that it was unnecessary but wanted to get the conflict over with so she could leave the hospital.

Naheema, a longtime vegan, had this exchange with her doctor in his office: he said, "You have to eat meat!" And she said, "No, I won't!" Her resolve faltered, however. Even though she did not have to contend with the kind of surveillance that had immediate consequences (discharge from the hospital was at stake in Jen's case), Naheema gave in "just in case," eating "very small amounts" of meat. When she began breastfeeding, she switched to sweet potatoes, which she believed would provide the necessary nutrients like Vitamin A. She described this dietary change as a "relief." By limiting their concessions, exceptional breastfeeders sufficiently preserve their self-concept and maintain their goals. They can remain privately critical of authorities' instructions while appearing to comply. Like one of those meme-style flow charts that all lead to one answer, these exceptional breastfeeders' decision-making always flows toward making sure their babies have what *they* think their babies need.

Drained of Power

Sometimes resistance feels futile. The new experience of having a baby and launching a breastfeeding relationship can be confusing, and there can be a steep learning curve. Jen explained her feelings of powerlessness: "When your milk first comes in, it's crazy that first time before you have a clue what your body is doing." Quiet coping can be the most sensible approach "before you have a clue." Breastfeeders may begrudgingly accept others' interventions, but this option is also exhausting. Some breastfeeders feel traumatized by "scare tactics" and victimized by interventions that subvert their goals. Formula feeders—and again, many, many exceptional breast-feeders also give formula—can be made to feel the same way for "resorting" to formula, which some segments of society designate as nutritionally inferior and evidence of inferior mothering.

Any of these caregivers may turn their disappointment inward, feeling like they failed as parents. Feminist scholar Rebecca Kukla writes of pro-breastfeeding ad campaigns that centralize the risks of not breastfeeding: "This shift in emphasis from giving benefits to avoiding harms will intensify the vilification of mothers who do not breastfeed and accordingly intensify mothers' own sense of indecency and inadequacy when breastfeeding proves difficult."[32] I wonder if these feelings of powerlessness may impact future reproductive behavior, perhaps shortening the duration of breastfeeding or contributing to the breastfeeder having fewer children. An alternative to quiet coping is to refuse this fate and take control.

BREAST MANAGEMENT PRACTICES

Mona fed her newborn "every two hours on the dot," as her doctor recommended. There are advantages to toeing the line by breastfeeding in prescribed ways—doing what the experts advise and what society can get behind. The two-mom form that Mona's family takes may flout norms, but her motherhood can be mainstream (at first, before difficulties arise). Likewise, breastfeeding in exceptional ways brings about certain political benefits in identity-making, social inclusion, and exercising one's beliefs and values. Some nonconforming breastfeeders recruit experts and turn institutions to their advantage by engaging select cultural scripts (e.g., science backs up breast milk as ideal nutrition, good mothers will do anything to ensure their children get the best) and by strategically applying pressure.

Consumer Power

Breastfeeders wrest some control over their bodies from medical service providers and institutions by brandishing their consumer power—demanding good service, assembling and directing their medical service team, shopping around for providers, and filing complaints. Consumer power is an element of class privilege.

It is this sort of privilege that afforded me the support I needed to breastfeed my son Leo. This effort began the day after his birth. He was screaming when I met him. My son was on his back, attached to monitors under bright fluorescent lights in a cacophonous room full of noisy machines and a labyrinth of incubators—some with hand-wringing parents hovering nearby—and busy, loud-voiced nurses. I could not wait to get him out of there. As soon as the sweet-natured hospital social worker finished her bureaucratic work with me and was safely out of earshot—make no mistake: she could bring my plans to a screeching halt and even stop the adoption—I asked to see the hospital lactation consultant. Having met her before, I knew her to be generous. She provides free consultations to breastfeeding parents who have their babies at other hospitals or at home. I explained conspiratorially that I'd lactated spontaneously upon meeting my first adoptive son and that I wanted to try breastfeeding the second. She lent me one of the coveted, powerful hospital-grade pumps and asked the on-call doctor to give me a prescription for domperidone, stat. Later, Leo's pediatrician kept up the off-label prescription and also provided a prescription for milk bank milk that I could purchase to supplement my own supply. They were all in violation of some policy or another. But nobody asked me any questions. Of course they wanted to help. To deny my requests would be poor customer service. My health insurance covers a group that calls me and sends me surveys to fill out after any visit to be sure of my satisfaction. It is a veritable "Club Med" compared to the local emergency room, in which I had occasion to wait in for six hours when one of my children needed stitches late at night.

Dorinne, a pediatric RN and thus herself an expert, had a starkly different experience when she encountered recalcitrant hospital authorities. They insisted on fierce adherence to their narrow policies, forbidding her to breastfeed or provide breast milk to her newborn. Dorinne and her doctor-husband found themselves at the mercy of this "archaic" institution—as she described it—because that was where the birth mother gave birth:

> They felt like allowing me to give her either my breast milk or even another donor's breast milk was equivalent to them giving the wrong medication to the wrong patient. . . . They wouldn't let me breastfeed her unless I was tested for a whole list of diseases that they came up with. We kept hoping that we would be out of the hospital before we would be able to figure out how to get these tests done and prove it. Just ignorance on their part and just being stuck in old school ways and just not being up to date on human milk and its importance.

This hospital was geographically and culturally distant from Dorinne's well-to-do urban life. She and her husband were livid. Ordinarily they could flash their credentials and expect better treatment. If they could take their business elsewhere, they would. Under circumstances that seemed hopelessly backward and ignorant, they had to be satisfied with submitting formal complaints and hoping for more widespread policy improvements.

Consumer power is not equally available to everyone. The working-class breastfeeders I interviewed could not choose their doctors. Anthropologist Dana-Ain Davis underscores the fact that professional black women may get no better treatment in hospital settings than poor black women.[33] Her research reveals that pervasive racism limits the protections that elevated class status confers to whites.

Good service extends to bedside manner. Young breastfeeding mothers complain of being treated rudely by providers who seem to assume that they will fail, according to Emie, who works with teen moms, and according to posts I collected from online breastfeeding support groups.

Some exceptional breastfeeders may demand emotional labor, though, as well as clinical expertise from their service providers. Valerie had four children, and after having had her fill of impersonal providers, she said "genuine caring needs to be demonstrated" before she would continue to visit them. Tayshia came to a similar realization through a process I think of as "experience contrast"—the shortcomings of a medical service provider, institution, or policy stand out in sharp relief against more affective, personalized care. When the hospital lactation consultant first came into the room, "she was in a rush, talking really fast, and then slapped the baby on my breast and left! . . . [Breastfeeding] just wasn't happening and I had to wait and wait and wait for her to come back. And then the nurses were coming in and saying, 'Why don't you just get some formula?'" Tayshia saw an acquaintance who happened to be a private lactation consultant. This provider was "heaven sent," an RN with medical knowledge, who also provided conversation, comfort, and reassurance along with a specific and effective protocol. This one Tayshia could recommend.

Team Players

The opportunity to choose medical providers and other supportive players goes a long way toward the ability manage them. Obviously, insurance coverage and/or extra funds to pay midwives and doulas and private lactation consultants help in this regard. Kadijah had the knowledge and wherewithal to seek out a midwife who agreed to "stay in the corner" unless she was needed. This cooperation helped Kadijah to have the low-key, independent birth she wanted and to start breastfeeding immediately after birth. She preserved the "natural" relationship with her baby by rejecting any and all interventions.

Private service providers may be better at respecting birthing and breastfeeding parents' preferences. Tara and Sandra witnessed the difference. The couple told me, "We've had experience with who you get when you are on public assistance, and we've had experience with who you get when you can afford a nice doctor. The nice doctor was fine and lovely and respectful of our relationship, and, like, no issues there." But when they needed to use doctors who accepted Medi-Cal, the public insurance in California, they had to correct a nurse on how to address them. The nurse refused to use language that respected the nongestational mother's role. Laughing, Sandra said, "She didn't apologize. Not like your nice, cozy, progressive, middle-class experience."

Some breastfeeders collaborate and collude with authorities to get their needs met outside of the official rules and policies. Kylie confided in her doctor about giving her baby raw cow's milk: "I didn't want to get turned into CPS [Child Protective Services] or anything for giving my baby something healthy. And when I told that to our doctor, she was like, 'I totally agree with you. I would pick your battles. You are not going to change people's minds. So I would just tell them that you have her on the soy formula.'" It almost goes without saying at this point: middle-class parents can bend the rules more easily than working-class ones.

Executive Decisions

Like those parents who treat their child's teachers like members of their staff—directing them instead of deferring to them as experts—some breastfeeders act like executives in charge of medical service providers. Connie, a breastfeeding comother of one child from Denver, carefully selected a team made up of individuals with quality résumés who passed muster in her rigorous interview process. First, she and her wife hired a doctor who was "a medical legend among Colorado lesbians" to manage their fertility care. They sought cultural competency in conjunction with medical know-how. (Rexi, a gender fluid parent who uses either "he" or "she," articulated a distinction between providers who are "immersed in queerness rather than nervously polite.") When it came time to breastfeed, Connie consulted expert-authored books written by and for lesbians. She purposefully avoided the traditionally heteronormative, sometimes dogmatic, LLL: "I feel like La Leche League is also militant in their stance: there is only one way to feed your baby. And that's difficult because as much as I'm not a huge fan of formula, I do believe it's necessary in some cases, and I think it can be discouraging for people when you are feeling so desperate about feeding your baby to be told, 'Don't do formula,' when you're thinking, 'How do I feed my baby?'"

Connie's politics as well as her individual needs informed her help-seeking strategies. She had sufficient social capital—friends in the know—to steer her toward high-quality options. She deployed the privileges afforded to a white, urban, educated professional to pave the way for a comfortable, accessible, and literally *manageable* mothering experience.

It can be much more difficult for other constituencies to have a full array of choices available and to successfully impel doctors and hospitals to integrate comfort into their care. Although providing emotional work around birth and breastfeeding typically falls to professionals who are lower paid—nurses, midwives, lactation consultants, and doulas in decreasing levels of remuneration[34]—their services may still be out of financial reach. (Many of the private practitioners offer sliding-scale rates, however, that take into account the patient's ability to pay. Some I interviewed even engaged in bartering arrangements.)

Many health care models expect family members to provide some of this care for free. The generational loss of breastfeeding knowledge is only one of the drawbacks that sets this strategy up for failure. There are limits on family members' time and skill. Strained relationships can also diminish the quality of care and support coming from family members. Dispassionate professionals can be more reliable.

But farmed out, divided care—wherein a single person has multiple doctors, a midwife, a doula, and a lactation consultant, each with a specific job to do—has its pros and cons. If the breastfeeder-to-be feels confidently in charge, she may be able to act as CEO, orchestrating and choreographing her care. The moment there is a snag, however—such as emergency surgery—the specialists may no longer function as a team. Conflicting advice and unwanted interventions can impede breastfeeding goals.

Taking Charge

The customer is not always right in medical settings. Some breastfeeders find themselves in direct confrontations. Harriet, living in the United Kingdom under a state-run medical system butted heads with her hospital-appointed nurse-midwife:

> I said, "She's feeding." And the midwife kind of looked at me like evidently I was this silly woman who didn't know the first thing about milk.
>
> And she said to me, "No, no, no. She can't be feeding; your milk won't be in yet."
>
> And I said, "She is feeding."
>
> And she said, "No, you are not listening: the milk won't be in yet." So I just took my bra down off the other breast, and I squirted the milk onto her shoulder.

The midwife is the accepted authority here.[35] But Harriet's body proved her assumptions wrong. As in this case, interpersonal struggles between patients and medical service providers around breastfeeding can become physical struggles. Harriet did not want the nurse to take the baby away since breastfeeding was progressing nicely. In this frustrated moment, she proved her point in a way that someone could conceivably portray as a near-assault (given the pathological fear of body fluids). Her statements were not sufficient for her to be taken seriously, a concern of many breastfeeders whose experiences do not jibe with authoritative knowledge.[36] Among the breastfeeders I talked with and observed online, it was not unusual for the provider to be cast as the culprit, foisting herself physically on the breastfeeder. Connie put it this way: "I heard stories of lactation consultants grabbing women's breasts and shoving them into baby's mouths. My initial response was indignant. How dare they touch your body!"

Social strains over breastfeeding play out dramatically in these memorable skirmishes. It was Jessica's husband who ran interference for her in the hospital. He physically removed a bottle of formula from a hospital nurse's hand to stop her from giving it to the newborn while Jessica slept. The nurse would not abide by his verbal objections—she cited policy and the need to get the baby fed as she continued—and so he had to block her. The nurse thought that she was doing her job—following written guidelines meant to produce certain measures for the medical chart, like number of feeds, ounces in (formula), ounces out (wet diapers), and, ultimately, infant weight gain. Jessica and her husband simply wanted the best for their baby, and to them, that meant breast milk. Choosing breast milk over formula, to many people, is a consumer choice, a parent's right, and a matter of bodily autonomy all at the same time. Jessica extolled her husband's courage in standing up for these rights. In their case, it was not an emergency, but sometimes the difference between breast milk and formula can be a life or death situation. Anthropologist Tanya Cassidy writes about her son who was born prematurely in Canada and died of necrotizing enterocolitis, a condition that newborns are more likely to survive if given expressed breast milk instead of formula.[37] At the birth of her second son—also premature and this time in Ireland—her husband pushed the hospital to acquire donor milk from a milk bank as Cassidy recovered from blood loss. They chose the hospital for its proximity to the milk bank and came armed with this plan should it prove necessary. Most parents cannot foresee the limitations of their providers. It took a devastating loss for Cassidy and her husband to approach the situation with such a degree of preparedness.

Risk Management

Jessica's difficult nurse speaks for a different set of values. She represents a large institution with policies often designed not to provide the highest patient satisfaction but to minimize liability and risk. Sometimes personnel transmit their risk aversion subtly. Nurses in a New Zealand NICU allow donor milk when they think the need is legitimate, or "medically necessary" (as in the case of necrotizing enterocolitis), but they remain uncomfortable with what they see as a risky practice.[38]

Risk is everywhere. Medical personnel may emphasize to the parents the risk to the baby's health in not accepting formula, partly because they worry about their jobs. Meanwhile, public health narratives[39] and probreastfeeding posters hanging on the hospital walls admonish parents about the risks of using formula.[40] Medical and legal risk narratives limit the consumer model as a source of power for breastfeeders.

Even so, the boundaries set by risk are not insurmountable. When Jeff, a gay adoptive father, gave his baby donated breast milk for a while, he and his partner suddenly thought to ask their pediatrician if there was any risk to this practice: "She kind of freaked because she realized that she never communicated to us that there was risk. She consulted with a pediatric infectious disease doctor just to talk about the risk and came back and said, 'Look, I mean the risk is so limited, but we're going to check [your baby].' A series of tests to make sure everything's fine. So he had an HIV test, hepatitis, and of course we're freaking out."

The prompt testing and the doctor's freak-out upset them initially, and such an event might be enough to stop many parents. But Jeff and his husband's desire to maximize the benefits to their baby by giving breast milk outweighed the slim likelihood of tainted milk. (A trusted doula friend vouched for the friends of friends who had donated to them.) Maximizing benefits may be, by definition, the flipside of minimizing risk, but this more positive spin preserved the couple's autonomy. They were acting as good parents by providing the best that they could.

Labor Power

At work, breastfeeders have even less power than they might have had as consumer-patients. Melanie's workplace story exemplifies the kinds of hassles workers have to deal with:

They didn't have a lock on the mother's room door, which I was like, "What?" [disbelieving] The very first time that I went in, I can't. I am kind of awkward because I had never [pumped] before. I had tried it at home a couple of times, and it was just like muh [uncertain]. And I knew I needed to pump at least three times a day because that is how often he was eating at home, and the second time that I was pumping, somebody walked in on me, and it was a busy hallway. And I was like, "What is this? Is this how pumping is supposed to be?" So I did a little research, and I found out that, by law, they are supposed to put a lock on the door. I went to the head of facilities and—he was like a sixty-five-year-old guy, and he was just, like, a dude. [Laughs] "Oh, great, I'm going to talk about my breasts with this guy." And he didn't want to put a lock on the door because the doors were nice, and he didn't want to ruin the doors. And I was like, "Oh, hell no." I actually had to go back to him with a copy of the law and explain to him that he was breaking the law by denying us this right. And eventually I had to say that I didn't want my coworkers to see my breasts, and then he actually believed me. He did eventually about a month later. I had to go through HR. It was a whole thing. I was like, "Really? Put a lock on the door, dude!" They weren't really open to the fact that I needed to pump, and I couldn't just put it off for a couple of hours. I just couldn't. I really had to fight for my legal right to use the pumping room on my breaks and at lunch.

Like other workers who need to breastfeed, Melanie had to invoke labor power and point to labor regulations in order to get what she needed. Even though Melanie possessed the sense of job security to advocate for her rights in the face of resistance, waving around policies was still not enough. She also had to withstand her personal discomfort in confronting the formidable "dude" who needed to actually add the door locks. Melanie did not want to discuss her breasts with this man but did it anyway for the sake of her hungry infant son. Her baby had some significant health struggles that made these efforts more poignant. Many would give up at this point. Melanie couched her request strategically in language that would make the custodian recoil. She counted on the truth nestled in the old joke that referring cryptically to one's "lady trouble" can stop any unwanted questions from male bosses, coaches, and teachers who do not want to know any more (presumably because they find women's bodily functions repulsive).

Leaves of absence to establish breastfeeding, pumping time and space in the work environment, and in some cases, the latitude to go off-site for breastfeeding are among breastfeeders' needs at their paid jobs.[41] Most postindustrial societies offer more generous accommodations than the United States, which lags way behind. Paid leave probably accounts for why breastfeeders in other wealthy nations may continue for a longer duration.[42]

Partly as a result of Melanie's bad experience, she changed jobs and experienced a big difference: "There were three mothers' rooms for a company of about 600 people, and then my other company, there were three pumping rooms for a company of 1,500 people. And there were locks, and there were actually comfortable chairs, and there was a whole system set up for reserving it." But this was a luck-of-the-draw situation. Employers who are not compelled to provide adequate accommodations often do not. Even when the laws are on the books, enforcement may be lax.[43] It can seem hopelessly out of reach in the context of U.S. politics, but if paid leave were more widely available, breastfeeding would be a much easier proposition, more babies would be breastfed and for longer, and it would lift some of the worries about timing of feedings and pumping sessions.[44] The freedom to determine one's own mothering journey seems unlikely in a world where being a woman is effectively a "preexisting condition," however.

COMPLIANCE AND COLLEGIALITY

These themes of uneven workplace compliance with breastfeeding laws, face-offs with unhelpful coworkers, giving up and changing jobs to better accommodate breastfeeding goals, and determined, uncomfortable self-advocacy appear again and again. Many skilled workers, especially those in male-dominated professions, complain about losing status when colleagues know of their too obviously "female" need to pump and breastfeed. The pumping room that Melanie finally got was an awkward space. People intruded by using it to make personal calls, and she once walked in on a pair of coworkers occupying the space for a furtive make-out session.

Breastfeeders who work in the military, law enforcement, and emergency services often feel isolated in their efforts as they maneuver in cultures that can be distinctively hostile to women. According to the nonprofit advocacy group Breastfeeding in Combat Boots, they have to negotiate policies and balance group needs—that is, "unit readiness"—with their individual breastfeeding goals.[45]

I interviewed Bailey, a firefighter looking for donated breast milk for her deceased sister's children. The value of teamwork that is integral to law enforcement and emergency response culture actually benefited her quest. She discovered a veritable bucket brigade of New England cops and firefighters who pass along donated breast milk to others within this community. Because of their vocations, she trusted their ability to follow protocols and did not need to know them personally to feel assured that they would safely handle the milk. Narratives about women's rights do not work well in this context, but conformity does. The participants in these milk-sharing groups see these parents as good citizens trying to provide the best nutrition to their children. Respected organizations like the World Health Organization (WHO) and the American Medical Association (AMA) back up breast milk as superior, breastfeeding as preventative medicine, and breastfeeding as a public health matter. These recommendations make for compelling arguments in masculinized, authority-respecting environments. But since the AMA and WHO now warn that informal milk sharing might be unsafe, these sorts of arrangements may be in peril.

Sometimes breastfeeding enhances a worker's status. Rexi, a transmasculine and gender fluid breastfeeder, told me about finally finding some common ground through the mothering talk she engaged in with other teachers at the high school where they all work. This experience strengthened Rexi's feelings of collegiality and belonging.

Whereas many breastfeeders cringe with embarrassment at having to store their milk and pump parts in a shared workplace refrigerator, Jen, an elementary school principal, discovered an unintended benefit: "The refrigerator is on the other side of the office. I constantly walk through, and parents are very unfazed by it. I actually think, to be honest, they kind of like it. I think it is something that they can relate to. . . . The school definitely has a grassrootsy kind of thing going on. A little crunchy, a little hippity-dippity in some ways." Instead of weakening her authority, as she once feared, her long-term pumping legitimized her status within the family-oriented alternative culture vibe. She was already in a position that commanded respect, and now she seemed like one of them too.

Breastfeeders working at lower-status jobs cannot count on their value to the employer (or their value to the clientele they serve) to ensure that their rights will be upheld or that their breastfeeding will be supported. Wait staff, store clerks, and other service workers who suddenly need extra consideration to maintain breastfeeding goals might find themselves left off of the schedule or given fewer hours with no stated reason.[46]

Obamacare guaranteed a free breast pump, a subtle hint to keep working at a paid job, but that is not enough to support breastfeeding needs. Those in feminized professions like nursing and teaching not only find it hard to time pumping breaks but also find themselves having to choose between nurturing their child and nurturing their patients or students. Confusion from others in the workplace may increase when someone breastfeeds outside the accepted norm, like continuing to pump at work past a baby's first year. Unfortunately, workplace compliance with regulations and policies that support breastfeeding seems to hinge on the breastfeeders' relative privilege and powers of self-advocacy. Not everyone can "win the good boss lottery," as Kimberly Seals Allers points out.[47]

GENDER "POWER"?

Food or medicine? Customs agents in Guatemala were bemused by a set of bottles packed in dry ice. Olivia, a prospective adoptive mother tried to get the donated milk across the border for her new daughter. She could not get them to understand, and the agents became so perplexed by her charades that they let her through. This sort of one-off occasion can be amusing, but it also reveals another strategy that helps exceptional breastfeeders get by. Especially where female bodies or gender nonconforming bodies are concerned, confusion causes discomfort—which produces the results they want.

Rexi, whose gender presentation varies, thought that having both a beard and large breasts was so discordant that most people never noticed the big pregnant belly; people strained to avoid staring. Nobody offered her a seat on the bus, but then again, nobody hassled her. Officials, who are compelled to notice uncomfortable things that they would rather not, like breast milk or perhaps an SNS under one's shirt, may want to get the interaction over with as soon as possible. There are too few social scripts for them to follow, so they look the other way to avoid making a scene.

Roxanne made a scene breastfeeding in church. Other women warned her that they planned to "tell the ecclesiastical leader to tell [her] to stop." They thought modesty should prevent her from breastfeeding in church, but the bishop—a man—responded that it was none of their business and gave Roxanne the go-ahead to keep nursing as she saw fit. Sometimes it is breastfeeders' praiseworthy compliance with gender roles—namely, immersion in motherhood—that gives them sway with authorities who allow them to violate other social norms. Breastfeeders occupy what some perceive as a mysterious and inscrutable other sphere. Authorities' discomfort and concerted ignorance, or their belief in deterministic gender divisions, may unintentionally favor nonnormative breastfeeding practices. Naming and normalizing these practices, such as milk sharing, may lead toward milk regulation. And though regulation (like paid leave) is necessary to ensure procreative justice, policies often tend toward limiting women's procreative freedoms.

ASSERTING AUTHORITY

There is yet another way for exceptional breastfeeders to open up more options: become experts themselves. They assert their newfound authority in a few different ways.

Our Bodies, Ourselves

"I do my research," Naheema explained. She read books, took classes, and scoured the internet for relevant advice on feeding and caring for her baby.[48] Many exceptional breastfeeders intensify their studying and their internet outreach when initial plans fall apart or when they want to engage in adaptive breastfeeding for other reasons. There is now a glut of information and support available compared to even seven or eight years ago. The new problem is sifting through contradictory advice.

The available experts-for-hire may not have the skill or the specialized knowledge to help in all situations. Mona regretfully described her doctor's limitations: "My endocrinologist said, 'Well, not all women can make enough milk.' And she proceeded to tell me her story about how she had to give her baby formula." Because her doctor's personal experience did not convince Mona any more than the medical conclusion, she went in search of a different answer without a guide.

Exceptional breastfeeders become experts on their own bodies and their own babies. Some get so immersed in the attendant research that they decide to pursue lactation or birth-related careers, whether paid or as a volunteer. The routes to expertise vary and may involve formal, accredited education, training for lay experts (e.g., LLL), abundant personal experience, or merely privileging one's intuition. Their authority remains at odds with some doctors, nonetheless, because even IBCLCs, professionally certified breastfeeding consultants, reside on the lower rungs of the institutional hierarchy. They cannot prescribe medicine or rescind doctors' orders. Knowledge offers limited power.

Working within the System

"Pull the literature to show me at what point was I at higher risk," insisted Rosemary when her care team escalated medical interventions during her first birth. A nurse conversant in medical jargon and the culture of biomedicine, she knew how to demand accountability in terms the authorities would understand and respect. She shucked the role of compliant patient. And she requested documentation, acting not so much like a customer-patient as an internal auditor, forcing the medical team to professional justification. It was not a matter of questioning policies but of enforcing them. Rosemary tried to rein in the machine of medicalization, but she did not question the whole regime. Susan Falls points out that milk sharers may be "questioning the hierarchy of scientific over intuitive knowledge" but asserts that their milk sharing is not "a rejection or dismissal of science or technology but rather a calculated, embodied engagement with it."[49] Formally trained professionals like Rosemary and IBCLCs tend to take this sort of moderate stance.

Mira presented something novel to her medical team. Her personal experience was what qualified her to school the experts. After some miserable, overly medicalized experiences with the birth and breastfeeding of her first child, she particularly delighted in sharing her unique knowledge with providers who had much to learn:

The nursing staff comes in, and they are like, "What the heck is that?" . . . "Oh my gosh, that is the coolest thing I've ever seen! That is so much more effective than the SNS." They were like, "Can we bring the NICU staff in?" I was like, "Sure, come on in!" I've got both boobs out; I've got the baby there; I've got the Lact-Aid [type of SNS] set up; I've got the entire NICU staff in there checking that out and poking at me. It was so funny. I was so totally thrilled because at least they know about this. If there is another mom that has the same problem, at least the education has now been there. So it was awesome.

She enjoyed a receptive audience—others have the opposite experience in medical settings—and instead of managing or coping with authority, she asserted it. She happened upon this role reversal accidentally, but then she embraced it as a way to contribute to future moms like her. Context is everything. That they were "poking at" her was just a fun scene, not any kind of unwelcome intrusion. Arguably, her adaptive breastfeeding is a variety of "biocompliance"—medical authorities approve of her embodied mothering practices. The SNS and donor milk provided a twist on that theme, but in this instance, it was not particularly unruly or defiant. As a middle-class white mother doing the best she can to provide gold standard care for her infant, she slots neatly into a familiar social role. She was not queering breastfeeding so much as she was advocating for keeping it going with the use of the proper tools. *Biodefectors*, described by Ruha Benjamin,[50] on the other hand, refuse normative compliance in scientific and medical situations. Medical authorities (and politicians) see some bodies as more problematic and pathological.[51] Mira had confidence in her body and in the staff's respect for it; hence she did not mind their clinical gaze. Her resistance came without opposition. By contrast, Sami, who is transfeminine, has to protect herself from this gaze because, for her, it is often hostile (at best, morbidly curious). She is not biocompliant in *her* adaptive breastfeeding.

Whether exceptional breastfeeders' authority stems from experience or formal training—or, more likely, a combination of both—these expressions arc toward the political. They retake some power, subtly and overtly critiquing the normative approaches to breastfeeding. For example, when adoptive parents use an SNS, they defy assumptions about who can or cannot breastfeed. At the same time that they comply with mothering standards, their practices call foul on the idea that mother-baby dyads are indivisible.

COUNTERMOVEMENTS

Some exceptional breastfeeders reject whole systems of control. Others embrace components of countermovements that fit more easily into their lives, their identities, and their politics. Whatever their beliefs and practices, exceptional breastfeeders still face layers of structural oppression. Sexism, racism, ableism, and homophobia benefit some breastfeeders and not others. A comprehensive survey of breastfeeding countermovements is outside the scope of this book, but I offer a few examples from the lives of the exceptional breastfeeders I interviewed to illustrate ways in which they may innovate from the margins.

Getting Crunchy

The breastfeeders I talked to, who come from all walks of life, cannot get enough of the word *crunchy*. It succinctly explains their exceptional breastfeeding choices. *Crunchiness* is what sociologists call an overdetermined[52] phenomenon; it emanates from many different (even opposing) social forces, any one of which could have produced this way of being known as *crunchy*.

So-called crunchy parenting—mostly associated with mothers—runs the gamut from droll, nominal participation in "natural living" fads to ardent, off-the-grid survivalism. It is a badge of pride, an insult, or an ironic label depending on who says it and the context. Just about any divergence from the established standards counts: home birth, breastfeeding, baby-wearing, cosleeping, organic cloth diapering, forgoing vaccinations, making baby food, homeschooling or "unschooling," alternative medicine, placenta encapsulation, and gentle parenting commonly wear the crunchy label. The trendiness of it all and the whiplash-fast commercialization of crunchiness—$55 Danish wool diaper covers anyone?—make it ripe for jokes. One internet meme goes, "We only eat local, organic food blessed by vegan unicorns." Clearly, crunchiness is steeped in class politics. "Mom shaming" abounds in crunchy circles.

Crunchiness purports to be liberating—and it often is insofar as it rejects medicalization and other authoritative oversight—and yet it is also aspirational. Being in the know—having the right products or engaging in up-to-the-minute practices—marks social class, or *distinction*.[53] Living up to a crunchy mothering ideal can be expensive, so knockoff versions of coveted crunchy products and dabbling in natural living help approximate the ideal.

(Organic) cherry-picking from crunchy options frees breastfeeders from taking on the whole identity, from embracing the left-leaning politics of it. Valerie, an engineer, evangelical Christian, and mother of four, distanced herself from "you know, the holistic living, the home birth people, the people who do the essential oils stuff." She proclaimed herself a moderate, saying, "I don't do any of that." She wore the label only because her extended breastfeeding appeared crunchy to her coworkers and because she spent "a lot of time reading and observing [crunchy] ideas." Valerie did not specify which crunchy ideas she liked and which she did not, but suffice to say, she was not drinking the Kool-Aid.

Crunchiness is not all that liberating in the sense that it is very much wrapped up in contemporary ideals of motherhood as the ultimate expression of femininity, of "momness." Jace, a transmasculine breastfeeder, recalled trying on a "crunchy granola mama" persona because it seemed required to be a good mother. Momness can be about looking the part as well as about acting it—by closely monitoring what chemicals come into the home or what foods and medicines go into the children's mouths or what materials touch the baby's skin. Crunchiness is burdensome by design—product marketing helps with this by demanding that choosy mothers choose the pricier organic versions of any product. The crunchy story fits in with the mother blaming so ubiquitous in American politics.

But being crunchy has value. The time, effort, and money that it takes adds to this value. Often, it starts with extensive research that calls into question innumerable mainstream assumptions. A lactation consultant gave Tayshia an article about how her diet affected her breast milk—the chief concern was mercury in the fish she occasionally ate. She remembered the process of getting crunchy: "I start reading more and more and more and learning all of these things. And reading how much chemicals had infiltrated our food system, and I realize, 'OK, everything has got to change.' I started learning about plastics. My makeup went away. I stopped wearing nail polish. Bleaches went away. Cleaning products went away. I started buying organic. Plastics went away. Teflon went away. [My husband] was like, 'We're going to be living in a yurt!' 'Maybe,' I said, 'but our toxic level is going to be low. That is what I know.'" Tayshia, repulsed by the bill of goods she had been sold by big industry, which was poisoning her family and profiting all the while, changed her entire lifestyle. She breastfed her daughter for four years, shared a bed with her for many years after that, and loved these choices. Being crunchy, for Tayshia and for many other parents, is a beautiful journey. The central concern is the child's health, but crunchiness also proves parents' dedication. And it is always an exercise of resistance against select mainstream messages that have political significance. Reject-ing formula can also be part of a larger rejection of environmentally destruc-tive farming practices, corporate profiteering, and inadequate food safety regulations.

Crunchiness encourages ritual. Exceptional breastfeeders, who are almost always crunchy by definition, even if they themselves spurn this identity, rhapsodize about their homemade baby care concoctions. Breast milk is an especially miraculous substance that can be mixed with oil for earaches, made into soothing soaps, creams, and frozen treats, saved in vials for eye infections, diaper rash, and acne. It is healthful and homespun to be crunchy. In a DIY world, crunchiness operates outside of rampant commercialization—until we start buying breast milk ice cream,[54] that is.

Crunchy people may distrust medical authorities, but they trade one kind of moralizing surveillance for another. Consider Kylie's process for making formula: "We just ordered all of the ingredients online, and then the recipe for the formula calls for cow's milk in addition to cow's cream. So we learned how to separate that ourselves, and it also calls for whey, so I learned how to make the whey myself as well. My mom was also very sup-portive, so she actually helped me do a lot of the legwork and research and order the products and things like that." She began with the word "just" as if the fix were simple, when it is anything but simple.

Even gaining access to the raw milk, which she did not mention in this passage, entailed its own labyrinth. Though she got involved because her daughter suffered significant digestive problems, making the formula became its own performance of maternal love—much like breastfeeding (or preparing a meal from scratch).[55] This is the positive side of crunchiness.

On the flipside, the crunchy code can be a lot to live up to, and it often mirrors medicalization in the exacting attention it requires. It reminds me of fake meat in the shape of chicken nuggets or burgers. Instead of just showing vegetables as they are, we attempt to make them fit into the exist-ing dining culture. Rejecting mainstream parenting but falling prey to the commercialization of "greenwashed" products that pretend to be environ-mentally conscious is equally superficial.

For the record, I encountered precious little of this latter attitude among the exceptional breastfeeders I interviewed. Their adherence to crunchy values was often pragmatic and rational. Aaliyah's family judged her nega-tively for breastfeeding "because of society." She went on to say, "And I did not care about society. Because that wouldn't make sense. Like I am going to stop feeding my child something that is natural and healthy to feed them something artificial that costs me money and then I have to worry about mixing? I am like, this breast milk is the perfect flavor, it is the perfect temperature; why would I do that?"

Taking on a "natural and healthy" orientation guided Aaliyah's subsequent choices. Crunchiness like this can be a touchstone to return to whenever doctors or family members or any other judgmental observers try to force their conventional ways on mothers. However much people (including the exceptional breastfeeders I talked to) may make fun of the "cult of crunchy" or critique it for its seeming lip-service resistance to powerful norms, it signals a shift in values. If this shift is uneven, it is because full-on revolution comes at a high cost to individuals' status and comfort.

Procreative Justice

"I was like no one in my community. No one knows about doulas and midwives and nursing like this except—I do not want to put anyone in a box—but privileged women get to afford something like this. That's usually the middle-class white women," noted Imani, a black mother of two living in Massachusetts. Most of her family members were not particularly supportive of her breastfeeding, preferring her to use a bottle like everyone else they know. None of her black friends, she said, even tried nursing. She told me that she had a hard time allowing herself to enjoy the benefits of breastfeeding and the "amazing, empowering labor and delivery" she had knowing that other women of color lack those opportunities. Imani wanted people who look like her to see her nursing and know that was possible. "Change the world maybe," she said.

And then Imani attended a retreat in Brooklyn for black women interested in birthing. There were doulas who were women of color walking by in every direction, breastfeeding their children uncovered, tandem nursing their active toddlers, chatting and supporting each other, and acting like it was all the most common thing in the world. She thought to herself, "Where have all you people been hiding?"

Imani explained, accurately, that African American women are dying while giving birth at five times the rate of other groups and that the cost of a private doula—whose services might reduce iatrogenic risks—is woefully out of reach for many women of color. She offers a sliding scale doula service that is urgently needed, and she says, "I have to do what my doula did for me, for other women . . . [who] probably wouldn't have one otherwise." It is very nearly a charity, as she realized that a hypothetical eighteen-year-old on her own could not pay the going rate—$3,000—for a home birth; by contrast, there are no out-of-pocket expenses for a Medicaid-covered, conventional hospital birth. "I'm not Ina May living on a farm," she pointed out. Though the denizens of the Farm lived in near poverty, they had social capital within the hippie countermovement. Many of the exceptional breastfeeders I talked to mentioned two of Ina May Gaskin's popular how-to books/manifestos: one on home birth and one on breastfeeding.[56] But some black home birth and breastfeeding advocates recently decried some insensitive remarks by Gaskin about how racism affects birth outcomes.[57]

The need for culturally specific support around birth and breastfeeding cannot be overstated. Black women have the highest infant and maternal mortality and the lowest breastfeeding rates in the United States.[58] As Acquanda Stanford deftly writes in her graduate school thesis, "Uncovering Imperialist White Supremacist Capitalist Patriarchy in Professional Breastfeeding Services: The Greater Complexities of IBCLCs,"[59] the main source of clinical support, lactation consultants, is overwhelmingly white. Women of color and members of the working class in general find themselves shut out of the prohibitively expensive, protracted route to this profession.

White feminism can be harmful to the needs of women of color in its privilege and tone deafness. Cringeworthy media headlines announce the anniversary of the Nineteenth Amendment with lines like, "It's been almost one hundred years since women got the right to vote!" But black women faced substantial discrimination in gaining access to the polls until the Voting Rights Act of 1965 (and there are still efforts to stifle their votes), and they were largely left out of the women's movement in the 1970s. Today, women of color continue to be left behind, black women being paid only $0.63 on the dollar (and Hispanic women only $0.55), compared to white women's average of $0.77 on the dollar. The larger reproductive rights organizations like NARAL (National Abortion Rights Action League) Pro-Choice America and the National Organization for Women (NOW) are run by white feminists.

But the SisterSong collective and the National Latina Institute for Reproductive Health, which both grew out of a black feminist caucus formed in 1994 at a pro-choice conference in Cairo, emphasize procreative *justice*.

This insistence on justice instead of rights expressly attends to fairness and access to procreative autonomy for women of color, trans people, and indigenous groups.

Some exceptional breastfeeders immerse themselves in a counter-movement apart from white crunchiness and more in line with reproductive justice, also called procreative justice (since we do not really "reproduce," as if children are facsimiles of their parents). I interviewed several breast-feeders who mother their children within a distinctly Afrocentric milieu that resists not only medicalization but also capitalism and patriarchy. They highlight sisterhood and African tradition, grounding their practices in an understanding of history (black granny midwives as original experts, black wet-nursing as politically charged legacy) and a skeptical approach to main-stream ideas about mothering.

Tiana's midwife practiced the same African Traditional religion that she did, a serendipitous discovery. When they first got together to discuss the coming birth, the topics ranged widely, covering all the body-related matters (including breastfeeding) as well as life in general. Tiana, who lives in Atlanta, entered motherhood in the embrace of an intentional commu-nity: "The good part about the midwife that I had, she built a community of moms. There were a lot of moms who breastfed for longer periods of time. It was not that big of a deal to breastfeed longer than a year; it was actually the norm in that community. Not in the outside world. Not in the outside community but inside that community, I saw so many moms doing it that I thought, 'Yeah, I'm going to breastfeed at least eighteen months.'"

Everything this group of mothers does defies popular expectations. They are black yoga teachers, massage therapists, and artists, educated and choos-ing to live on the fringes economically and politically. They seek authentic-ity; that is what defines them, not validation from the dominant culture. Together, they build new norms to follow that might or might not be in line with what is happening on the outside.

Embracing a countermovement vis-à-vis breastfeeding does not require total immersion in an alternative way of life. It probably helps: Aster, a Latina mother of two and a Rastafarian, lived virtually off the grid—I traveled down a series of bumpy dirt roads to meet her at her home—subsisted within an underground economy, and disbelieved all big media and government-sourced information. Her breastfeeding choices almost needed to be countercultural to maintain her politics.

Still others, like Kadijah, found it possible to live on multiple planes. In addition to her "primal birth," she breastfed with no cloth cover for three and half years and donated her milk, all to the mild chagrin of her more conventional family members. She did all of this with the support of a grass-roots network of like-minded friends, whose narratives and practices were, in many ways, outside the reach of institutional authority.

"Our milk is revolutionary," reads a tweet and Instagram post from December 30, 2016.[60] The message, sent to various reproductive justice organizations, includes a black fist and the hashtag "Kwanzaa." It is breastfeeding as political rallying cry, bringing black women together for collective strength.

Revitalizing Resistance

Winnie had always been a perennial believer in breastfeeding. She amassed strong opinions over the course of decades volunteering as an in-home breastfeeding counselor. Time had been her teacher. "Who is scaring these women?" she asked indignantly, noting women's increasing germophobic reluctance to leave the house with their newborns. (During our interview, she laughed at herself and frequently checked in with me to see if she was "driving [me] crazy" with her soapbox soliloquies.) While Winnie acknowledged that formula was sometimes necessary, she said that doctors are "marketing to themselves" by suggesting that a bottle of formula here and there could make nighttime easier. In her opinion, doctors should counsel mothers that it is normal for breastfeeding to be hard, for babies to wake many times in the night. Mothers, she averred, should expect this work and should be unafraid. Breast pumps are no "magic" gizmos but another kind of shackles in Winnie's view. She explained that she wanted to bring back mutual child rearing and breastfeeding support systems that she and her hippie friends modeled in the 1970s.

Breastfeeding, currently in vogue in mainstream white America, never went away for Mormons. Kiki, a mother of eight children, left the religion but maintains the belief in maternal divinity:

It's not anything that I've done any research around. I take mother's intuition seriously. I really value it. I hold it in very high esteem. I think it's one of the great duties of being a mother, that you have that. I noticed the children who are breastfed tend to be more pliable, if that makes sense. Whereas children who are formula fed seem stiffer. . . . Of course, all of the latest research comes out and says that you should [breastfeed], but I just figured God gave us breasts for a reason. Why go and try to make something better than that?

She followed her intuition to such a degree that when she dreamed up an epic family road trip, she took her children out of school and traveled the country in a van for months with no set plans. Her extended breastfeeding, tandem nursing, and milk donations are hardly the most radical aspects of her mothering. But they do add vitality to her political and cultural expressions. Even if she no longer subscribes to church doctrine, Kiki still espouses its rejection of state meddling and its embrace of mothering autonomy—motherhood being the exclusive, independence-streaked realm of women.

Breastfeeding is always a political act in the contemporary West. For exceptional breastfeeders, whether they espouse breastfeeding politics, come to embrace them, or simply live them intrinsically, they disrupt the status quo. We should listen to them. Their social positions and their political stances, as well as their specific obstacles to their breastfeeding goals, color their experiences with authorities. Breastfeeders need policies and regulations to support their goals but with a significant caveat. Oversight that is not broad-minded, sensitive, and flexible will only damage caregivers' freedom. Centering procreative justice on the actual experiences of real breastfeeders and bottle-feeders—who may or may not be women, who may or may not produce milk, and so on—is the path toward improvement. Like exceptional breastfeeders, we need to resist unchecked medicalization and pathologization of female bodies and breastfeeding "problems" and question the essentialization of women as mothers and mothers as women that is so much a part of the legal, medical, and educational doctrines. Political lessons learned from exceptional breastfeeders could guide changes that would lead to increases in breastfeeding initiation and persistence rates, maternal satisfaction, and other measures of public health. Such improvements are only worthwhile if they are driven by the breastfeeders themselves.

5 · BUSTING BINARIES
Embodying Otherhood and Motherhood

"A baby breastfeeding is an undeniable affirmation of our root-edness in nature." This quote, attributed to venerable environmentalist David Suzuki, adorns the web pages and social media profiles of many a breastfeeding advocate. Also "undeniable" is that breastfeeding is a bodily experience shot through with gender essentialism, including debatable assumptions about females being closer to nature.

Breastfeeding can also be a powerful site for queering and questioning essentialism. Exceptional breastfeeders, who by definition are already bending the rules, actively queer breastfeeding just as they normalize new and forgotten practices.[1] Not so long ago, breastfeeding reinforced the marginality of political radicals (like hippie "earth mamas"), religious minorities, and poor women. Now that breastfeeding is the middle-class ideal, complete with the celebrity endorsements and the baby-friendly hospital initiatives, people raise eyebrows when they discover that a mother is choosing not to breastfeed. Exceptional breastfeeding complies with some social prescriptions but also disrupts the gender/nature ideals that buoy these prescriptions. Breastfeeding can be about performing feminine motherhood as expected, or it can be about resisting that very discourse. What is interesting is that sometimes, incongruously, it can involve both.

FEMPOWER

"Breastfeeding is the single best experience of my life. Giving birth was really great, but breastfeeding over a period of years was really empowering. It was a time when I felt really connected to my body and feminine power," recalled Latisha. Breastfeeding is the ultimate embodiment of femininity for some women. Interestingly, Latisha's "connection" is not with her baby but with herself. As a black woman for whom breastfeeding reclaims stolen "feminine power," it even exceeds the wonders of pregnancy and birth. This becomes an almost tangible force as something lost and regained and now deployed in service of Latisha's liberation.

For parents via surrogacy, adoption, or fostering and for mothers who endured disappointing or traumatic births, breastfeeding may signify a singular opportunity to connect on that physiological and metaphysical plane commonly known as bonding. I feel like I bonded with both of my children, one breastfed and one not. There are many ways to establish that closeness. For some, breastfeeding fosters feelings of emotional closeness and a physical symbiosis. Breastfeeding my son made *me* hungry; his cries made my breasts fill with milk. In turn, the smell of my milk triggered his instincts to root and suckle. The milk satiated him, and its nutrients did their work growing his little body. Breastfeeding involves physiology, but context and social relationships make the experience. (Sex works this way too.)

Did I get in touch with my feminine power with breastfeeding? I may not have thought of it in those terms, coming from a different standpoint as I do, but I can certainly relate to the sentiment. I share Latisha's affinity for breastfeeding.

Gwendolyn, a mother of two, located her breastfeeding self within an even broader network: "This person came from nothing, and somehow I ate bananas and salmon, and this body grew inside of me, and now there is milk flowing through my breasts, and it's nourishing them and making them fat and pudgy and helping their brains grow. I am not in control of any of this, but I'm witnessing it happening through my body. So it connects all women. And all mammals. Throughout time. The fact that you are doing this: that's really profound."

I can pretend to scientific objectivity here and draw some functionalist connections: breastfeeding serves a manifest, practical function in providing Gwendolyn's children with calories and securing each child's psychological sense of trust and security. It "connects all women," as she said. So perhaps breastfeeding also holds the latent potential of binding women together in their collective imagination, a phenomenon that anthropologists call "psychic unity."[2] A public health audience might appreciate a concrete, testable set of suggestions from these findings—such as marketing ideas to improve breastfeeding initiation and persistence rates. (Advocacy materials might try accentuating tradition or the miracles of the body, for example.)

I could instead "go native," as anthropologists say, and revel in breastfeeding's profundity like Gwendolyn did. It's an appealing antidote to the cold medicalization of women's bodies. But what I wish to promote here is an analysis that (1) takes exceptional breastfeeders' experiences seriously and (2) recognizes that breastfeeding bodies and gender interact in various ways that are not mutually exclusive. A single breastfeeder can call up widely accepted gendered meanings of breastfeeding and can subvert them at the same time. One significant finding from my research is that gender essentialism itself can be queered by breastfeeding.

Olivia had an experience that was inextricably biological *and* social when breastfeeding made her breasts bigger. Laughing, she said of her body, "It's more womanly looking than I ever have been. I feel like a Renaissance painting." She felt like her lactating breasts temporarily magnified her femininity, and for Olivia, this experience was fun. Maybe she was inviting a sexual male gaze. Or maybe the bigger breasts merely improved fashion aesthetics (a different woman, Roxanne, suggested to me that her breast size increase helped her fit into clothes per their design). As the curvy bodies revered in Renaissance paintings do not exactly match the current standard that fetishizes thin or "strong" bodies, Olivia's body goes against the norm. The change in some breastfeeders' bodies is "fun," a recurring—but by no means universal—motif among the study participants.

Gender assumptions around breastfeeding allow it to serve as proof of identity and relatedness. This is the case for Shawn, a "boyish" lesbian, who identifies as Latina but is read by other Americans as black (she emigrated from the Caribbean). As a lesbian, a gender nonconforming person, and a person of color, she is put on the triple defensive by the historical and contemporary mistreatment of mothers belonging to these social categories. Society continually calls into question their motivations and their fitness for motherhood, and these social messages impact Shawn's identity as a mother. She said of breastfeeding, "It makes me feel like a real mom." It is real because it is an ongoing, thoroughly embodied, daily practice that requires sacrifice, as Shawn implies. And "real moms" make sacrifices (or so the story goes).

Breastfeeding for Shawn (and Latisha, for that matter) is also akin to a revitalization ritual, such as when a threatened cultural group—like some Native Americans—publicly performs forgotten ceremonies. Shawn said that breastfeeding established and reestablished her indispensability as the mother. "I don't want to feel like an outsider," she explained, going on to say, "It's something only I can provide." Her queer gender presentation and sexuality put her legitimacy as the true mother at risk in the public eye, but breastfeeding's feminine biopower validated the relationship.

Exceptional breastfeeders use this essentialist discourse that breastfeeding is feminine while also chipping away at gender assumptions. They do this strategically, if obliquely. Jace's complicated relationship with breastfeeding is telling. A transmasculine, pansexual member of a polyamorous romantic triad, he experienced both *physical* struggles and emotional discomfort with what he saw as biological imperatives. He complied with—and resisted—breastfeeding-related social forces:

I have not had any physical, medical interventions [for my gender transition]. I basically held off on that so that [my son] could continue nursing because taking testosterone limits the milk supply. I went through what they call my "crunchy granola mama phase" with my daughter, where I was trying to fulfill this idea I had of what motherhood was supposed to be. I wore long dresses, and I was just trying very, very hard to fulfill this certain image I had on what I should be as a mother. And with my son, I kind of had this epiphany: I do not have to do that. I can be a good parent without fulfilling this ideal I held up before, and it would be better for everybody if I was just myself, and so I kind of went back to dressing the way I did when I was younger. Which is masculine and just presenting myself more authentically as me.

Breastfeeding's relationship with motherhood, being a wife, body dysmorphia, sexual identity, and touch aversion all come into play in Jace's search for authenticity. By trying on the role of the ideal breastfeeding mother by dressing the part, and then rejecting that role, Jace recognized that his constant discomfort was due to gender dysphoria. The traumatic physicality of breastfeeding, which involves such an obviously female part of the body, and the very femininity of the performance, he felt, clarified his true gender identity: "Sometimes [breastfeeding] got to be a little too much for me, and I would be really hard on myself for that because I was just, like, a horrible mother because I did not like it and things like that. But with my son, I have been able to set better boundaries, and that helps me manage. Sometimes I don't want to be touched, but I still want to nurse him, so I just kind of set boundaries, like he is not allowed to mess with my other boob while he is nursing and things like that." Breastfeeding led to Jace's self-discovery. With his former way of thinking, Jace felt like he was a bad mother because he did not like breastfeeding (he was supposed to feel "motherly" nursing his babies and did not; ergo, he was a "horrible" mother). This suggested to him that he was not truly feminine. And it is this essentialist mumbo jumbo around breastfeeding—that mothers should be feminine, that breastfeeding equals motherhood, that mothers should love breastfeeding—that eventually aided in his active rejection of his gender assignment.

He eventually worked it out. Jace continued to breastfeed, rhetorically and performatively separating the two ideas of breastfeeding (being a good parent) and femininity (being a real woman). He literally set new boundaries, disallowing his son to play with the other breast, for instance, which let Jace breastfeed while still respecting his own gender-related physical limits. Jace went on to tell me of another boundary: he looked forward to having his breasts removed as soon as his son weaned—not something Jace wished to rush for the three-year-old's sake but an event that was sure to happen soon on its own. At that point, he said, he could "finally have done with them [his breasts]" and look on his robust children with pride, knowing he nurtured them well.

THE SECRET LIFE OF AS, BS, CS, AND DDS

> There is a big stigma behind the boobs. . . . You have to be dedicated because it is not easy and picture-perfect like you would hope it would be.
> —Kerry

"Useless saggy old things." "Living food." "Beautiful." "Rawhide-like and deflated." "Not up to par." "Working and able." "Big and fun."

Breastfeeders described their breasts by appearance and function positively, negatively, and neutrally in my study. Australian researcher Monica Campo conducted a focus group study and found that some breastfeeding mothers wrestle with maintaining their independent senses of self when their breasts seem not to be their own anymore, whereas others enjoy giving in to a greater feeling of connection.[3] This connectedness, she points out, citing Barbara Katz Rothman,[4] does not jibe with our cultural preoccupation with individualism.

There are wide-ranging ways of experiencing this contradiction. Several breastfeeders told me they had never really thought about their breasts much, that they were "milk delivery vehicles" or "feeding devices." Cricket noted that she would not be devastated if she found out she had to get a mastectomy; breasts did not matter to her once she was no longer breastfeeding. In these cases, breasts may not have ever meant much to their identities to begin with. Other breastfeeders I talked to missed their once-perky breasts but figured any loss of appeal was a fair trade for a healthy, happy child.[5] A small percentage of them wanted reconstructive surgery to restore their breasts' appearance and, by doing so, hoped to regain their figure and their sexual attractiveness. Mira had her "lopsided" breast reconstructed. Her young daughter, who knew of Mira's discomfort with her breasts' appearance, said, "I hope I don't get boobs like yours, but if I do, I know you will help me nurse."

Some strictly separate breasts for breastfeeding and for sex. Kadijah refused to date until her toddler weaned: "I suppose it was, like, sexual reasons. I suppose I didn't want to have my breasts all tangled up like that." Others have no such qualms. They have a "dual role," explained Kiki, who nursed her children and her siblings' children *and* enjoyed her breasts during sex with her husband. This dual role might be a significant source of liberation if it were more easily accessible for breastfeeders. The social context in which nursing is supposed to be done in private, in which breasts are under the medical gaze as nutrition and medicine dispensers, in which nursing bras look utilitarian rather than sexy, reinforces Kadijah's conservative approach, not Kiki's more liberal one.[6] Of course, Kiki already gravitates toward contrarian thinking in all aspects of her life. But as exceptional breastfeeding becomes more commonplace, the resulting diversity in experience may lead to less constricting attitudes about breasts.

The Dynamic Duo

Jace's experience vividly underscores breastfeeding as a versatile gender performance. Breasts are dynamic in their meaning and function, quintessentially bound to gender embodiment. For many who have them, but especially for exceptional breastfeeders, breasts are revered *and* troublesome body parts that have an almost independent life of their own (hence all the anthropomorphizing ahead). Sometimes they betray us, refusing to produce as expected or becoming painfully engorged. Other times, as we have seen, they confirm our worthiness as women, as mothers, and as providers. Milk donors delight in their breasts' productivity. Lactating breasts work hard and redeem themselves from lifetimes of being too big, too small, too asymmetrical or unattractive, or too attention-getting.

Because breasts are so highly sexualized in America, they sometimes stir up trouble in partner relationships when their use changes. Kadijah appreciated that her ex-partner remained supportive through her three and a half years of breastfeeding despite her lack of libido. She said, "My constant nursing left me very sexually not wanting to do anything. And that was difficult for our relationship." For others, robust, milk-filled breasts enhance the romance. Realistically, as a breastfeeder and baby nursing relationship goes on, surpassing the newborn months of intense care and frequent feeding, the experience changes. A married couple I am friends with told me a story about a time when the breastfeeding wife insisted that her body knew the difference between toddler nursing time and sexual time with her husband. The punchline? The milk sprayed him in the face unexpectedly, and the two shared a good laugh.

Whether we want them to or not, breasts mark identity, changing others' perception of gender and gender roles. Consider the symbolism of lacy, push-up bras contrasted with functional-looking nursing bras. In a different sort of double bind, the sexy bra celebrates one kind of femininity and the nursing bra another. And lactating breasts may even change one's gender status in the eyes of the public, such as when a butch-identified or transmasculine person who ordinarily binds their breasts suddenly cannot hide them.

Carefully tended breasts may refuse to behave. They have a tendency to become more unruly with lactation and breastfeeding. Such was Mona's experience:

I love my breasts. Before I got pregnant, they were my asset. They *are* my biggest asset. I love them. I have tattoos on them. I call[ed] attention to them with some of the clothes that I used to wear before I became a mom—very low cut—and I even had pierced nipples at one point. And since then—I still love my breasts—I wish that they would work better. [Laughing] But since I've been breastfeeding, they've gotten bigger, which has been nice. And I enjoy having breasts, so I can imagine if I ever got cancer or anything and had to remove them, that would be very devastating.

Mona said that she loved her breasts three times in this passage. They were integral to her self-presentation and to her identity. But they betrayed her when they did not perform as she wished with breastfeeding. She felt inadequate as a mother when her supply proved insufficient. Her breasts did not "work" well enough, but at the same time, they were bigger and she enjoyed this aesthetic. Her breasts' misbehavior may have impaired the validity of her gendered motherhood, but her value as an attractive woman slightly made up for it.

Kiki recalibrated the meaning of her breasts depending on the situation, an effort that did not always turn out to her satisfaction. She recalled, "I think it was a love-hate relationship. I thought they were hot. I had great boobs. My breasts. However, at the same time, I hated attention for them. If somebody else was attracted to them, I didn't like that at all." She wanted to determine how others perceived her breasts. Her cousin's husband would not allow Kiki to nurse their baby when she babysat because he thought it was weird. She became upset that "they've been so sexualized, that the beauty of them nurturing a child, like he couldn't see beyond the sexualism behind it." To her, they were sexual only in context, and she demanded the prerogative to determine when her breasts were to be seen as nurturing and when they were "hot." She could "see beyond" their sex appeal, and if others could too, we would not have to debate the right to nurse in public.

Bosom Buddies

And yet breastfeeding breasts have relationships with others beside their owners. Kadijah said of her preschooler, "She is four and a half now, and she still tries to get my breasts. She has a very close attachment to them. They are her friends almost. Like she needs to touch them. She always talks about them. They have their own relationship."

Jeri and Allie, co-nursing mothers, joked that "we will never look at each other's boobs the same way again." When Jeri claimed to not care about hers, Allie interjected that Jeri's breasts are particularly attractive and that Jeri knew and enjoyed this fact. Jeri conceded the truth of her wife's counterclaim but added that she liked having a more "athletic" physique. As with many couples, Jeri's breasts mean one thing to her and another to her mate. Their discussion not only illustrates the dynamism of breasts' meaning and identity-making but also reveals how breasts' significance gets negotiated with others.

Moving the Spotlight

A popular blogger, "Ms. Wright," a young black mother and breastfeeding advocate, posts high-quality photographs and videos of herself online pole dancing in a bikini with her baby on her back and exercising with her toddler nursing. These posts always provoke numerous conversations in the comments sections about what it all means. Someone—often a man—accuses her of being an exhibitionist, and others rush to her defense. Her point is akin to Kiki's view: breasts can be attractive, nourishing of babies, *and* sexual. Ms. Wright's activism is performance art. She pushes the public, especially the black community, to rethink the compartmentalizing and disembodiment of breasts. Breasts may seem to have a life of their own, but in truth, they are never apart from the whole person.

Latisha was on a mission to convert the public perception of breasts even as she grappled with her own views on her own breasts: "I would just like more knowledge in the black community that breasts are not a sex organ. That is secondary. They are not just there to flaunt. If that's what you want to do, that is your choice. But they were given to us because we are mammals. And all mammals produce milk to feed their young. Period. And that is basically my standpoint on that. It is frustrating." Her frustration extended to lingering internalized oppression; she struggled with needing to feed her baby in public but knowing that her family members would think she was being immodest. Latisha "check[ed] herself," asking, "Why are you doing this?" to be sure that she was not showing off. She then affirmed her intentions and answered herself: "To feed your baby." Support from her community, she realized, would make breastfeeding much easier. She also took a certain kind of feminist stance by refusing to impugn women who *were* "flaunting" their breasts. Instead, Latisha requested the moral space to nourish her baby without everyone looking askance. She drew on the mammal trope in order to declare her behavior part of the rightful order of things. Feminists shudder at such language because it dismisses women's humanity and autonomy. Women are complex and much more than mothers, much more than mammals doing what we are "naturally" designed to do. Latisha would likely agree with this critique, but she invoked an existing essentialist cultural logic in order to shut down debate about her choices.

Reembodiment

When breasts change, so does the self-concept of breastfeeders—sometimes. Carena, a black, single mother living in Atlanta, put it this way: "I think there's a certain level of how you own yourself and how you see yourself as more than physical property. So I mean, I would like them to be a little bit more firmer sometimes, but aside from that, they are no longer like, 'OK, they are just way too big.' And now like, 'OK, they did a great job!' It is more than just accoutrements."

She loved how her breasts finally had a purpose other than garnering unwanted sexual attention or making it difficult to find bras and clothing that fit. It made Carena feel better about her body and herself because her breasts became "living food." She said with amazement that she had "become whole." The breasts were no longer an accessory but "life itself." This experience adds up to gender empowerment. Women are not accessories. Women are not property. It means even more for black women, who live with a legacy of being "property" in an absolute, literal way. Through breastfeeding—however it gets defined—breasts have gone from disembodied property to reembodied. Carena owns herself now, and that self is newly whole.

Zest for the Breast

Like a weird relative, for all their recalcitrance and irritating idiosyncrasies, lactating breasts can be fun. But the fun to be had must be on breastfeeders' own terms for them to reclaim their breasts in empowering ways. The probreastfeeding documentary *The Milky Way*[7] lingers on a scene in which a breastfeeding mother playfully squirts an arc of milk into the pancake batter she is mixing. The filmmakers highlight the scene to normalize breastfeeding and breast milk and to place the power with those who are doing it.

Breastfeeding in the United States and many other parts of the West is not so normalized as to be perfectly routine. Illogical taboos about body fluids and breasts persist. But it is the very strangeness of breastfeeding that makes it fun for some. Kelly said, "It was totally fun. All of a sudden your body making these weird secretions . . . especially when you are waiting for a baby, seeing how much milk you can make." At this point in our interview, her wife interrupted her. "Marybeth [Kelly's wife] says it was not fun." After a beat, Kelly amended her earlier statement: "Pumping was not fun." Obviously, the labor of it, from pumping to sleepless nights, put distinct limits on breastfeeding's entertainment value.

Joanie, a butch lesbian mother, had this to say about breastfeeding and the body: "It was just kind of remarkable. Not fun in like a sexy way but just like whoa! Bodies are crazy. But they could just change that much. It's so great. We talked often how good it is that you don't have to be in charge of any part of the child-growing process. Like, 'Oh, we have to feed the liver now?' I would have forgotten to make the liver, and lots of things would have fallen to the wayside. Your body just is amazing." Joanie is not one of the breastfeeders who usually enjoys having breasts; when not breastfeeding, she wears chest-flattening sports bras. Her breasts were merely tools for feeding babies. But her experience shows another pathway to empowerment.

Instead of feeling freshly reintegrated with her body like Carena did, Joanie's embodied power came from the enjoyment of discovering the body's capabilities. With virtual sentience, her amazing, remarkable, crazy, fun body operated on its own accord to grow a child. Joanie's whimsical role as appreciative bystander obscures the very real bodily labor of breastfeeding. But this sort of framing allows breastfeeders who lean toward a masculine identity (like Joanie and like Kelly above) to keep a comfortable narrative distance from their breasts. Having this sort of fun also balances out the drudgery. Having fun queers breastfeeding in the sense that it flirts with the stigmas. For many, "normal" breastfeeding demands modesty. But squirting milk and inducing lactation and being bosomy while butch can be all about disregarding modesty and reveling in nonconformity.

EXCLUSIVE BREASTS

Not everyone likes to share. "He doesn't touch my milk, and that's the way I like it," said Susan about her husband. She did not want him to rearrange the bags of milk in their freezer. The ownership of breasts—and, in some cases, breast milk—may come under contention during breastfeeding, and it can change the duration and quality of the practice.

Quality Control

In Susan's case, this exclusivity was about managing her body and maintaining quality control over "her" milk, some of which was donor milk. Her proficiency in handling the milk and breastfeeding with a supplemental nursing system (SNS) was a source of motherly pride. The mother in a family typically takes charge of the family's nutrition and the organization of the kitchen work; to some degree, Susan's preferences were probably an extension of these norms. Still, being the "only one" who can breastfeed one's baby is one of the most cited unintended benefits of breastfeeding among the study respondents. Susan's body could not produce all the milk, but she could perform a strong maternal role by taking charge of the milk and its delivery.

Ownership Matters

Kiki first thought that her husband's interest in her breasts after she gave birth the first time was "weird." But when, in desperation, she sought his help in dislodging a clogged milk duct by applying suction, she did an about-face: "He became my savior instead of this person who wanted to invade my mom thing." The realization that she could apply different meanings and functions to her breasts was liberating. She still owned her body. Remember, she wanted to control others' perception of her breasts, but she was able to let go of exclusivity.

Invasion of a breastfeeder's "mom thing" can be an abiding concern. Some breastfeeders worry less about any awkwardness around their breasts being sexual than on maintaining an exclusive mother-baby dyad. When someone says they are committed to "exclusive breastfeeding," or EBF for short, they mean that they do not use formula. But one of the consequences of exclusive breastfeeding is that, presumably, nobody else is feeding the baby. Especially as it goes on for many months, this dedication can be a disappointment to grandmothers and partners who had expected a bigger role in feeding the child and thereby access to bonding time.

Some partners are OK with breastfeeding out in the open at home but cannot deal with it in public, at least at first. They may jealously demand modesty. Yesenia's conservative police officer husband reluctantly supported her breastfeeding in public and pumping at work until the child reached age two. At that point, they argued about it until she appeared to give in. In reality, she began nursing their child not just in private but in secret until the child neared age four.

"How many times are you going to take your breast out?" asked Kadijah's mother. Many grandmothers want their daughters to conform to conventional rules of decorum. They also want to protect the men's sensibilities. Alice said as much: "I found myself cringing a couple of times. I was like, 'Sweetheart, aren't you going to cover yourself?' And she was like, 'Why?' She will nurse uncovered in front of my daddy, her grandfather. . . . Even with all of the years of breastfeeding, I still usually take my cues from my spouse—my ex-husband and my current husband. They are not comfortable with anyone seeing any part of my breast, so I think that is probably the reason why."

Not only is breastfeeding a private matter that some think should happen at home and not in public, but the breasts are not for just any family member to see. The baby, the intimate partner, the supportive grandmother—these folks get special access. It's not unlike cultural practices that keep a daughter hidden until marriage—wedding veils are a vestige of this tradition. The sight of breasts is particularly controversial because they signify sexuality, which does not jibe with the cultural image of appropriate motherhood. The concern about fathers seeing their daughters breastfeed extends the "boundaries of touch" proscription that exists because of entrenched social anxieties about sexualizing one's children.

Time and Attention

Breastfeeding sucks energy and time. Aster tandem nursed her two infants, and she felt overwhelmed by the attendant "hormones." She said, "Although it is so positive and enlightening for the children, you disconnect a little from your partner." She experienced a bodily urge to establish the relationship with the babies. Of course, Aster also had to contend with the flagging energy and touch fatigue—the feeling of being "touched out" with constant physical contact—that many breastfeeders experience. Getting back to her intimate partnership motivated Aster, and others like her, to put an end date on breastfeeding. Eventually the breasts would be "back in the game," as Sabine put it. Her breasts were too sensitive for sexual play during her nursing days. (For others, the breasts *lacked* sensitivity, which diminished their role in sexual activity.) Time and attention given to the breastfeeding babies temporarily cut into the time and attention available for partners. Long-term breastfeeding may further strain the partner relationship.

Limits on available time and energy may become heightened when the breastfeeding is no longer exclusive to the family. Spring worked this out by designating her milk donations for medical emergencies only: "It's something that I'm doing intentionally, and it is taking away from my family and my own time and my own life. You know, I'm glad to be doing it. It's important to me. I think it's also just me being . . . one of those rational types; I just want something kind of concrete to go off of for picking who I was going to give milk to, and I decided that the criterion that was important to me was that the baby needed the milk and not—I wanted that to be my basis—and not the mother." It is already difficult for women to meet the expectations that their bodies and their breasts be sexually available to their partners and also be dedicated to intensive motherhood. Spring could make sacrifices to both ideals in order to help a stranger's or acquaintance's baby but not to help a mother who should be able to find it in herself to provide adequately. Spring was unwilling—because she needed to be present for her own family—to give so another mother could enjoy the luxury of "peace of mind." Spring said she did not want to become unwittingly complicit with a low-supply breastfeeder's lack of maximum bodily effort. Her preference here is EBF for all but in the absence of that possibility, then at least exclusively breast milk—to a point. Spring subscribed to the prevailing expectation that a mother's first responsibility is to her family. Even if she lends herself out for work, or for some other pursuit like milk donation, her time, her attention, and her physical presence belong to her family.

Toddler Demands

"I want boob!" Kerry's toddler yelled in the grocery store. It is "real subtle and discreet breastfeeding," she deadpanned. At a certain point, many nursing little ones begin to take ownership of the breastfeeding breasts, reaching into shirts, talking and wiggling and sticking feet in faces while nursing, demanding the breast like they would a toy or a pacifier or a banana. It becomes up to the breastfeeder to set limits if they feel comfortable doing so. Lanie said, "I think the beautiful thing for me nursing that long is that it does create a relationship where you have to connect and check in with each other. There were times when I didn't want to nurse. So what does that look like? And how did she appreciate that where she could get her needs met in other ways? And then we would come back to nursing. And it became this beautiful mutual relationship and not a place of me meeting her needs exclusively without conditions, you know? I definitely was part of the relationship." Lanie had to teach her little girl to consider her mother's needs too. Breastfeeders who extend breastfeeding into the toddler and preschool years have an opportunity to renegotiate their bodies as at least partially autonomous. The societal assumption is that breastfeeding is really all about babies. That Lanie even had to say that she was "part of the relationship" proves the point.

Some breastfeeders choose to wean when the experience gets to be too demanding on their bodies or their lives. Cricket realized that her only technique for consoling her daughter was nursing; she weaned the girl at age four in part so that her husband could do some of the work of comforting. She felt that the father-daughter relationship improved as a result. Cutting off access to her breasts stretched the dyad bond to make room for other caregivers. Cricket casually invoked medical authority by telling her daughter that doctors "turn off the milk" when kids have their fourth birthday. Counting on her daughter's undeveloped sense of time, Cricket left the house for a few minutes and returned announcing that the milk was gone. (The child was present during parts of our interview, and she did not remember weaning, only that breastfeeding was "yummy!") Cricket's creative lie preserved her relationship with her daughter by not turning weaning into a drawn-out struggle, a negotiation, or a matter for debate. Cricket also told me that she wanted her daughter to view weaning as a "societal expectation," something that everyone eventually goes through.

Other nonconfrontational weaning tricks, like putting Band-Aids or bad-tasting creams on nipples or wearing tight clothing, which make breasts more difficult for toddlers to access, count on the child to simply give up. Tayshia put a positive spin on weaning with a "bye-bye nursies party" for her daughter (some breastfeeders make cake like a birthday celebration, while others may invent rituals such as a special song). Like many breastfeeders,

Tayshia felt ambivalent but, ultimately, wanted to get her "body back": "We are just so mass-producing our lives. So for me [extended breastfeeding] is all part of our soul cooking. It is just that nurturing, that deep, deep nurturing. I nursed until she was four. . . . I don't know that she was done so much, but I was like, 'I don't think I can do it anymore.' I was just really kind of tired. I just felt like I really wanted more of my body back."

Tayshia noted "subtle pressure" from society to wean, pointing out that her daughter was especially tall and so seemed even older than her four years. Tayshia's body belonged to her daughter, who did not want to wean, and to society, who thought she should stop nursing. Her desire to get her body back was about reintegrating herself with her body and her breasts. It would also be a better body than it was before for having provided milk (and for having healed from past sexual abuse trauma).

Tandem nursing triggers more claims on breasts and breast milk. Sometimes siblings resist sharing with the new infant. When I nursed my new infant, my older son, only fifteen months at the time but an early talker, would protest indignantly, "I'm the baby!" as he pointed at himself. Olivia's experience was different: "Since I had worked so hard to lactate for her, I would let her nurse until she quit on her own. And I was coming to grips with tandem nursing, and then after he was born, she wouldn't nurse, and I had severe engorgement. And I begged her to nurse. And she just said, 'No, those are for the baby.' And she never nursed again."

Because an infant's nursing pattern and suction strength differs from that of an older child, many breastfeeders nurse their multiple children at separate times, making for many sessions in a day. Ironically, breastfeeders may feel more disengaged from their own bodies—in terms of autonomy—at the same time that they are more beholden to demands on their bodies than ever.

Attachment Equality

"Attachment equality" refers here to the insistence that neither partner take a privileged role in caregiving in order to equalize each parent's opportunity to build a relationship with the child. Breastfeeding, as a part of doing gender, can make a difficult nexus of identity performance, family building, and caregiving. Marnie, an adoptive mother of one from New York, identifies as a high femme lesbian. Her partner disdained the practice of inducing lactation and breastfeeding:

It's actually been, like, our biggest bone of contention. My best guess and what I have heard her say is that she doesn't understand why the baby would need to nurse if he could get his nutrition from a bottle, number one. And then she says, "What does that mean about my bond with the baby if you're doing this to foster attachment? How does that affect the attachment that I have with him?" So you know I did point out to her that she does technically have the same equipment and could also breastfeed, but she is transgender and didn't think that was very funny.

Marnie's transmasculine partner did not want to be the odd man out. Since breastfeeding, in their case, required inducing lactation and formula supplements, she (her pronoun preference) could not see any good reason to do it. She suspected Marnie's breastfeeding would effectively drive a wedge between the child and herself. Marnie's gender presentation fits more within the mold of idealized femininity, and breastfeeding further embodies maternal femininity. Her partner's breasts, by contrast, seem to challenge a masculine self. But just because she was more masculine did not mean she wanted to default to the dad role. In conventional imaginings, fathers are not quite as "close" with children. The queerness of their family building is put at risk by dropping into traditional gender roles. Marnie was able to reject this line of thinking, but because her partner was not, they fought. She wept during our interview at this turn of events. Breastfeeding meant a great deal to Marnie, so she sought support from others outside of her intimate partnership. Still, she did not nurse as often as she wanted because of her partner's preference, and weaning was prematurely on the horizon in her view. The result was that Marnie did not feel fully in possession of her own body and her own breasts.

Thomas also spoke to the idea of attachment equality. He and his husband mixed their sperm for an at-home insemination with a surrogate. Though they could tell by looking at their boy which of them was the genetic father, they chose not to emphasize it. Thomas very briefly considered using a milk delivery device to simulate breastfeeding:

[My husband] did not consider the device—I don't want to speak for him, but my guess is he would not have been [as] comfortable as I am with the idea of the baby sort of comfort nursing on me. That sort of freaks me out a little bit.

But I did consider some of the attachments. But then I thought that that is just sort of crazy. To me, the big issue is the eye contact when a baby is feeding and the touch issues. So as we were feeding him, that is really what we focused on. The eye contact and the talking and the touching. That was our way of sort of bonding.

Queering the male body in this way turned out to be beyond the pale after a little consideration. The fathers could bond to a sufficient and satisfying degree by finding other ways to simulate what they felt breastfeeders accomplish. They followed the socially prescribed steps toward bonding, substituting as needed. Their "way of sort of bonding" was as similar as possible to breastfeeding. Thomas and his husband did not compromise on nutrition, as they provided donated breast milk in the bottles; they delivered these with skin-to-skin contact in the baby's early months to foster attachment and to help the baby regulate his body temperature—which doctors identified as a bit of a problem for their baby. Just like when they mixed their sperm to get pregnant, the two matched their feeding and cuddling in a way that equalized their relationships with their son.

Our society fetishizes breasts and, arguably, breastfeeding as well. Multiple stakeholders lay claim to how they are seen and how they are put to use. The choices to be made and the conflicts and compromises that ensue usually evoke the duties of mothers. Various efforts to make breasts *exclusive* seem to always reinscribe gender boundaries.

REPURPOSING

Disembodied breasts, by contrast, may serve the opposite purpose. Some breastfeeders draw a stark line between gender and breastfeeding. Thad, a transman, explained, "I can feel close to my kid in many different ways. It wasn't that. It was functional—to make sure he had enough sustenance." He experienced his breastfeeding not as a tender, motherly practice but as "utilitarian" and solely for the purpose of providing nutritious calories. "I had a set sitting there. Might as well put them to use," he added. But one need not be transgender or butch to disassociate breastfeeding from the emotional and from the feminine. Valerie, a heteronormative, cisgender mother of four, insisted that breastfeeding was far from a "spiritual experience" and that there was none of that "super special bonding" that everyone talks about. Instead, it was simply ideal nutrition, delivered efficiently. It had its nice moments, she agreed, but so did ordinary cuddling. Clearly, not everyone agrees that bonding from breastfeeding—perhaps "extraordinary cuddling"—provides intimacy so intense as to be threatening to other parental relationships.

Some breastfeeders I interviewed distance femininity from breastfeeding by emphasizing breasts as tools or as a source of food or medicine. Some breastfeeders also experience it as a mammalian function or something to be endured. But social scripts do not always line up well with individual experiences. Breastfeeders create their own accounts, but that does not mean other people will get it. But breastfeeders who are already socially marginalized in some way, perhaps by being queer, have practice with being transgressive.

Cyborg Breasts

Breastfeeders often see themselves as milk machines. Many mean this as a joke or indicate that feeling this sort of disembodiment is but one facet of the experience. But for some folks, like Jace, who makes the machine analogy explicit, it is integral to identity. To him, breasts are a "piece of equipment attached to my chest." "I have a very utilitarian view of my own body. It is, in fact, not exactly conventional in terms of bodies and gender," he explained.

Breasts as tools function as "vehicles to deliver milk," as Thad put it. They provide "storage capacity," according to Rhonda, a single bisexual mother. They are "all-purpose parenting tools" for Roxanne, who has multiple views on breasts. The contraptions that make adaptive breastfeeding possible—the pumps, the SNSs, the nipple shields and nipple shelves, the low-flow bottles and nipple attachments, even milk-measuring phone apps—add to this cyborgification.

Function over Form

Breastfeeding breasts are "magic tools" for soothing tantrums. And they are a nutrition delivery system. Some breastfeeders cite these purposes either as vindication for breasts' otherwise annoying existence or as reasons to power through any unpleasantness with breastfeeding.

Tara, who is genderqueer and co-nursed her child with her partner, never really wanted breasts and was glad they "finally had a purpose." Originally, she did not intend to breastfeed but did so because her wife ended up with low supply. It was a happy accident that doing so made her breasts meaningful. Notably, it did not make her feel more feminine, just functional.

Sherry also learned to appreciate function over form but in an entirely different way: "I liked my breasts a lot less until I started nursing. I think I sort of started to see them as utilitarian, especially my big droopy right breast. I love it for all the milk it produced for all these babies and my babies. I want to have a little party for it when I wean. [That breast] made so much freaking milk, no wonder it looks like a deflated sack."

Whereas Tara did not want breasts at all because they failed to support her more masculine gender identity, Sherry wished hers were more "attractive." Her breasts were always asymmetrical, but the difference became more extreme. Thirty-nine-year-old Sherry said one breast looked like it belonged to a nineteen-year-old, while the other was depleted. But her breasts' performance exceeded all expectations, giving her a "massive" forty-pound toddler and allowing her to donate milk and to nurse friends' babies. That she wanted to have a party for the good breast that did not look as pretty is a testament to the power of a metaphorically disembodied appendage to "do gender" in an affirming way instead of reductively. Think of the Trump-like reduction of women as "pussies" available for grabbing and the mass movement response of wearing them, symbolically and knitted, on millions of heads. Sherry reclaimed her gender power by breastfeeding with "imperfect" breasts. The healing comes from thinking of them as utilitarian, a perhaps counterintuitive benefit of disembodiment. It is not scientists, doctors, or advertisers who are separating the person from the body part (for them to study, treat, and use for marketing purposes) but the breastfeeders themselves who are refusing to let a body part diminish them. Breastfeeders conceive of their breasts as tools to distance them from gender or, alternatively, to affirm gender.

Mammals Suck[8]

Rita, who pointed out the irony of being a midwife who cannot get pregnant, always knew inducing lactation was possible. Years ago, her roommate's dog spontaneously nursed two kittens they brought home. She planned to breastfeed the child who was her soon-to-be adoptive placement. Rita found solace in "Mother Nature's" ability to adapt in this way and placed herself within that web of life. Inducing lactation is not artificial. It is natural.

Alice joked that she is the "family cow" because she nursed her baby and her daughter's baby. The cow cliché connotes production (a lineup of udders attached to sucking devices), wholesome tradition ("Milk! It does a body good"), and dumb, domesticated subservience. Jen said, "There was a time at the very beginning when I didn't have milk supply. You are literally like a cow in a pasture. They [the babies] are just, like, *at* you nonstop. [Laughs] Because they are trying to increase the milk, they just keep sucking." In this comparison, a cow's body is not her own; it exists to produce milk for others. Even while they are aware of their bodies more than usual since they have to stop to nurse, to take in many extra calories, to manage supply, and to rest accordingly, breastfeeders' sense of bodily autonomy falters. Alice and Jen enjoyed this absurdity because they knew breastfeeding was temporary.

Jen gave some agency to the infants whose sucking makes her like a cow. But in other cases, references to mammals remove all agency from both breastfeeder and nursling. Some other phenomena emerge if we compare breastfeeders to mammals in general instead of specifically to cows. First, identifying as mammals connects breastfeeders to nature. It is a prime argument against using man-made formula manufactured in profit-driven factories and administered with insufficiently designed bottles that attempt to simulate breasts and nipples. Breast milk is nature's "perfect" food, in this way of thinking, and nature is thought to be much smarter than fallible humans.

In 1987, Margaret saw a sign at the gorilla enclosure at the zoo that indicated that their babies wean around age three; "See, Mom!" she said, pointing. If gorillas extend breastfeeding, why not humans, she reasoned, trying to convince her mother that long-term breastfeeding was natural. In crunchy thinking, natural means pure and right. And popular views of science assume that nature is self-correcting. Some breastfeeders harken back to nature to tie breastfeeding into a universal feminine maternity. But some gender nonconforming breastfeeders view their lactating breasts as androgynous, like a dog's or dolphin's milk glands that provide sustenance but do not reinforce femininity.

Second, breastfeeding as mammalian behavior puts physiology in power. We stand back in amazement watching our bodies perform astounding tricks.

A January 23, 2017, op-ed piece in the *New York Times* touted research that suggested that a lactating body produces different quality of milk for male children than it does for female children. The exact compositions are still sketchy, but researchers note differences in fat content (higher for boys) and calcium richness (higher for girls) by the child's sex. This sort of research—from the study design to the interpretations of the findings—naturalizes gender boundaries to such a degree that sociologists like me will suspect confirmation bias. This is just one recent example in a burgeoning science of lactation physiology and breast milk chemistry. It seems that infant saliva—that is, "retrograde milk flow," also known as "baby spit"—causes a lactating body to produce specific immunities that pass into the milk,[9] that hormone messages passed in milk cause female infant cervical cells to proliferate for later reproductive maturity,[10] that stress hormones in milk predict a child's temperament,[11] and on and on. (See anthropologist Katie Hinde's blog for a more exhaustive and up-to-the-minute list.[12]) Let nature do its job, the champions of breastfeeding might say. They can point to such work to show that we have only reached the tip of the iceberg in proving the breast is best—in an ever-narrowing definition of ideal breast-feeding. One conclusion could be that infants should get their personalized milk directly at the breast from their gestational mothers. Of course, critics of "lactivism" will say that such positions alienate those who use formula (or donor milk, for that matter).

Beyond all the usual controversy, the emphasis on physiological feats also has a disembodying effect. Exceptional breastfeeders who induce lactation and high-producing milk donors may sense their bodies acting of their own accord. Harriet, for instance, felt strangely honored when she met a milk bank employee who, not knowing she was speaking to the donor, waxed on about the "ooh, very rich, very creamy milk" that Harriet had been donating. Harriet told me that the characterization seemed very cow-like and she felt like her production of top-quality milk was involuntary, but she said the comment left her feeling proud nonetheless.

For many breastfeeders, the body just doing what it is supposed to be doing—or committing a betrayal by not functioning "properly"—feels largely involuntary. Along with respective doses of pride and shame, breast-feeders may also observe the process as a rupture between body and mind. Depending on who is doing the observing and interpreting, the breast-feeding body might confirm essential femininity or the act of breastfeeding may be a separable function, having nothing at all to do with the breast-feeder's gender identity.

CONSIDERED QUEERING

One way a breastfeeder can be "exceptional" is to breastfeed while queer. Some LGBT breastfeeders directly engage with the gender meanings and the performance of breastfeeding because it is so obviously coded as female and feminine. Nongestational comothers and those who identify as more masculine than the norm may be particularly aware of the ways in which their breastfeeding flouts these presuppositions. The result is a diffracted array of overlapping experiences. These range from reconciling dissonance, concerted dissociation of breastfeeding from gender, accepting contrast, deliberate queering, and defiant normalizing.

Reconciling Dissonance

"I am really surprised to find myself doing it at this point. I identify as pretty genderqueer, so the whole femininity of breastfeeding is a little strange to me. It is not something I identify with usually, and I've never had an easy relationship with my breasts," said Sandra. She and her partner both nursed their baby, sharing the work and the joy of it all. But Sandra noted, "It feels weird to be on the masculine end of the spectrum and breastfeed and attract weird attention if you do it in public."

Sandra's body dysmorphia was not something that her immediate queer community seemed to understand, though her wife was supportive around the issue. Other butch and transmasculine breastfeeders in an intimate online group provided her with much needed "focused support":

> Specifically having it acknowledged that I might feel a little bit strange on the masculine end of the spectrum, or at least butch end of the spectrum and breastfeeding. And then there's also just like practical things like nursing cups and what kind of clothing would be comfortable for us to wear from a gender perspective but would also be practical for nursing. Those two parts. It was super identity-confirming, that there is this dissonance in my breastfeeding experience and then just this other part where, "Hey, you can wear a button-down shirt and put a panel over it."

When still pregnant, Sandra's wife suggested that they both breastfeed. Sandra shifted her initial "No way!" attitude when her wife encountered low supply problems. Getting support from others who understood and could articulate the discomfort helped her keep breastfeeding through the gender weirdness. It was particularly remarkable that the practical advice—what kinds of shirts to wear and where to find comfortable nursing pads—most affirmed her butch identity. She could breastfeed in a butch manner if she wore the right clothing. It takes effort to sew panels into button-down shirts, but members of her support group have made and disseminated tutorials to spread the word. Breastfeeding can disrupt a nonfeminine identity—just as having trouble with breastfeeding destabilizes some normatively gendered women's status as "real women." But if a breastfeeder can reconcile the seeming dissonance, breastfeeding can also be done in a way that preserves a more masculine identity.

Dissociation

Let us consider Jace's position once again. The experience of breastfeeding helped him come to the realization that he was transgender, and he viewed his breasts as "equipment." But he went further toward disentangling gender and breasts: "I have never really had a problem with using my breasts for their intended purpose. Once I am done with them, I do not really have any use for them, though. I do not really see them as a part of myself exactly. . . . My breasts are useful, but once I am done with them. . . . I do not have any other use for them at all . . . as far as my social image of myself as a male."

Recall that Jace planned to have his breasts removed and then to embrace a body that more closely matched his gender. Similarly, Thad began binding his breasts after concluding breastfeeding and was on a waiting list for top surgery (breast removal). He too circumscribed his breasts' function temporally and practically for breastfeeding and nothing else. Breasts feel so gender constricting that they felt compelled to have them removed.

Yet these two men consider them tools with a purpose. Breasts doing the job of breastfeeding do not have to be more feminine, despite the fact that many people look at it that way. These stories show how breastfeeders' turning breasts into removable accessories dissociates breasts from conventionally embodied femininity.

More feminine breastfeeders may take this tack as well to free themselves from self-blame when breastfeeding does not go well or when breasts do not look as conventionally attractive as they may wish. Feminists rightly critique disembodiment of female parts as dehumanizing. But when the individuals with breasts make these distinctions for themselves, it is a matter of preserving their identities. Some transgender people and some disabled people talk about ignoring parts of their body or experiencing them as "phantom" or "ambivalent" rather than biological realities.[13] This discernment is important to understanding how rhetorically disembodying one's breasts—they are machines, they are mammalian parts—differs from essentialism. They are not saying that breasts are just milk makers but that, *for them*, thinking of their breasts as useful replaces the gendered meanings of breasts. Breastfeeding feminine women who happen to have low milk production may insist that these parts that "don't work" (referring to their breasts) cannot detract from their status as good mothers.

Accepting Contrast

"They are big. They are in the way. They are obvious. But, eh, they're OK," said Rexi about her breasts (with unintentional poetry). Her relationship with her breasts started in junior high and came to a head in her twenties:

> After college, when I started getting more into the queer community and started playing around more with gender, there were times when I thought it would be convenient if my tits were smaller and I could bind them or look different, getting men's clothing to fit how I want. But never enough discomfort that it was worth it for me to do anything about it, like consider surgery or hormones or anything. I occasionally wear sports bra[s] that would flatten my chest a little bit, but I am a D cup so, really, you know, I have tried on a binder once or twice, and they just look like I'm lumpy.

She did not mind that her "tits" did not conform to a masculine standard. Breastfeeding had little effect on her already-flexible gender identity. Devin, who identified as "fairly butch," articulated a parallel sentiment: "I'm accustomed to being a little hard to read and having boobs. . . . [Laughs] That might be something that if I was younger I might try to fuck with a little bit. I might try dressing more butch and really mess with people and have obviously feminine and obviously masculine characteristics together, but I don't really have the time or energy for that anymore."

Both have reached a time in their lives where they have already contended with their breasts and their bodies—Rexi and Devin were both gestational parents who experienced pregnancy and childbirth—and came to the conclusion that their masculine identities do not preclude their deeply embodied participation in procreative activities that society deems feminine. It is telling that Devin did not have the "time or energy" to publicly confront the perceived contrast; they did not make breasts gender-irrelevant, but at the same, they were merely indifferent to making sense of them. Both Devin and Rexi intentionally "play[ed] with gender" in their formative years, but this identity-making was no longer a priority by the time they became parents. They understood that their bodies confused others, but their focus on first-time parenthood took precedence.

Deliberate Queering

"They all think that it's interesting and that it's wonderful and a little bit exotic and pretty cool that I can breastfeed," remarked Tara, a genderqueer parent. She was talking about the reaction of her friends and family to her inducing lactation and breastfeeding with her usually masculine-appearing body. The emotional pain wrought by society's rejection of one's body, identity, sexuality, and legitimacy as a parent can be resisted, countered, or "fucked with," as Devin described it, in liberating ways.

Exceptional breastfeeding can be a protest of social strictures like gender roles and gender presentation. But its real performative significance happens around its role in parenting. Even though Tara's community loved the queerness of her breastfeeding, she herself felt more ambivalent: "None really know that it's kind of a mismatch for me and how I feel about my body. I've spent most of my adult life not with an easy relationship with my breasts because I'm just not that feminine. They're kind of big [now], and so it's odd for me that they're front and center and that I'm using them in this hyperfeminine way. Everyone else just thinks, 'This is great. This is cool!' There's no catch. It doesn't even click for anyone that it is weird for me."

Her bristling at being the poster child for queering gender serves as a reminder of the personal costs of being on the front lines. None of the gender nonconforming, gay, lesbian, or otherwise queer respondents I interviewed or observed online seemed to be motivated to breastfeed by

performing difference. They breastfed to care for their children, and negotiating their queerness was a by-product of that process. Tara described the
experience as "odd," "weird," and "a mismatch," not as any kind of purposeful challenge to gender norms. Breastfeeding, for her, was not meant to be
identity work or the political statement that her friends wanted it to be.

This reality contrasts with online chatter about gender nonconforming
breastfeeders by outsiders. In an effort to be more inclusive in their care,
some birth workers and lactation consultants recommend gender-neutral
language like "pregnant person" instead of "pregnant mother" or "pregnant
woman" and "breastfeeding parent" in lieu of "nursing mother." There has
been a backlash. In 2015, a self-described "gender-critical" group of midwives known as Women-Centered Midwifery sent an open letter to the
Midwives Alliance of North America decrying the latter's use of gender-
inclusive language in their revised "core competencies" for direct-entry (lay)
midwives. The critics claimed that neutral language that aimed to include
transgender birthing parents effectively neutralized women. They saw pregnancy and birth as an important source of women's power that should be
celebrated rather than obscured. Proponents of this critique—often part of
the trans-exclusionary radical feminist (or TERF) movement—also participate in online discussions of breastfeeding. They insist that a man cannot have a baby, that birthing and breastfeeding make one a woman. These
activities are exclusive to women, they argue, and transgender folks are sta-
tistically insignificant and/or are probably having psychological problems.
One midwife and trolling commenter writes, "Disassociating [sic] from
your sex and feeling dysphoric at its mention is definitely not 'well.'" Some
go so far as to argue that gender-inclusive language is "antifamily." Queer
parents may not *choose* to enter this political fray. Like most parents, they
just want to care for their babies.

Defiant Normalizing

The more frequent, mundane, and mainstream queering practices
become, the less queer they remain. Breastfeeding has become expected
for parents, so much so that gay men like Thomas, Jeff, and their husbands
acquired breast milk and simulated breastfeeding as best they could. Even
as they are queer and breastfeeding—very broadly defined—they conform
to parenting expectations, though gender factors into the experience. Providing breast milk to their infants and cuddling them skin-to-skin does not

feel like any threat to their masculinity (although Thomas's husband recoils at the idea of suckling because it *does*—and perhaps because it brings up discomfort about unfounded portrayals of gays as pedophiles). Queer breastfeeders along the gender continuum have disparate negotiations around the sexuality and femininity of breasts and their relationship to normal parenting.

Butches breastfeeding, for instance, is not yet an everyday scene. Some in the queer community can hardly wait for its "queerness" to pass, as the following conversation between Sami, a transfeminine mother who identified as a soft butch lesbian and her femme wife, Amelia, illustrates:

SAMI: I'm not feminine. I don't think of being a parent as being inherently feminine. I find it annoying, that "Butches and Babies" Tumblr, where everybody is cooing over these masculine women having a baby because like, "Surprising, right?" Because masculine people aren't supposed to be nice to babies.

AMELIA: So if they are, it is like a bonus.

SAMI: It's like a bonus. It's sexist, right? This idea that dads or masculine women or whatever, that there is something nonparental about masculinity. It is just sexist. So I'm not like, "Oh, I'm a mom now, so I should be like a pretty lady."

AMELIA: You *are* a bit more of a lady now.

SAMI: It's concurrent with becoming a mom that the way I present myself to the world has evolved.

AMELIA: I don't think that when people see you, they see that you are gay. You just have short hair.

Sami's gender and sexual identity are ambiguous to others. She was transgender from male to female and has a slight physique and augmented breasts. Until recently, she did not often wear dresses or make herself up in conventionally feminine ways. Her short hair was more of an indicator of butchness in some communities than others (she used to live in Los Angeles where long hair reigns for women). She exercised next level queering in rejecting breastfeeding and parenting as feminine pursuits. Sami let gender wash over her in the sense that she observed herself presenting in a more feminine manner but did not want to make any explicit connection to mothering.

Sami accepted the contrast without overanalyzing her gendered existence, and she also endeavored to normalize her parenting. She communicated a sense that breastfeeding, while a matter that requires some attention, was really no big deal, or no different than what anyone else does.

Breasts can be a salient part of a queer identity separately from being part of queer breastfeeding. Marnie pointed out wryly, "'Femme Mama' is not such a big thing." She explained that accentuating her breasts was all about "dating and being hot. And it is certainly not about motherhood." It is not a fetishized category for a femme (usually meaning an LGBT person who presents as feminine) to be a mother. They are distinct aspects of feminine identity.

The gendered embodiment of breastfeeding feels different from different gender standpoints. Shawn, who enjoyed a delightfully active nursing relationship that entailed unexpected positions, tickling, and wrestling bouts with her active toddler, calls herself "boyish," but she does not fixate on being thorough in her masculine presentation. She questioned her friend who cannot separate masculinity from good parenting practice—that is, breastfeeding: "If you are having a baby, you cannot get more womanly than that. Why would you not breastfeed the baby when that is what's best for the kid? Are you afraid of the image that is going to be put out there? 'Oh, this boy is breastfeeding a baby.' That takes away your cool points for being the stud, the masculine? . . . I don't care if you wear your pants below your knees, sagging and all that—if you have a kid, you were a woman." Shawn suspected that folks like she described might have some good reasons for rejecting breastfeeding, but she could not fathom them off the top of her head. She wondered why they could not continue to compartmentalize more effectively if they were going to embody pregnancy and childbirth, already coded as ultrafeminine. Here, she seemed to agree with the TERFs (who now take umbrage at this acronym). Shawn's gender fluidity allowed her to be womanly in one way and boyish in another. Other gender noncomforming parents feel less comfortable with this seemingly extreme code-switching.

And still others radiate indifference. Because Marybeth's breasts have never been important to her gender self-concept or to her sexuality, breastfeeding did not impact those aspects of her identity. A partnered lesbian who co-nursed her adoptive child for four years, she said her gender was "unremarkable either way." I asked her how she thought of her breasts after having breastfed for a long time. Her reply was, "I didn't really pay much attention to them before, and now that I'm not [breastfeeding], I don't pay any attention to them now either. [Laughs] That wasn't really part of it for me. You know, I am fine with them."

Mothering the Milk

Jeff considered how the breast milk donated to his son by up to twenty women amounted to something of a maternal influence: "A piece of them has helped shape who he is, and he's such a well-adjusted kid. He's comfortable in big group environments with anybody and everybody, and I think so much of that is the energy that came from these women. Not just the antibodies but the actual energy that flows through their body and into his."

Once more, breast milk is not just food and medicine. Sometimes the meanings move into the mystical. Here, I focus on the maternal embodiment of "liquid love." This approach resists medicalization, commercialization, and risk stories by making milk into something that regulators cannot touch and that factories cannot reproduce.

The Milk Makes the Mother

For Eve, whose baby died soon after birth, pumping and donating her milk allowed her to continue in the role of a mother, albeit to a limited degree: "The thing that I didn't expect was that it was really healing for me to be able to donate milk because I felt like I didn't get the chance to be a mom to my son, but being able to make milk and donate it to other babies in the NICU [neonatal intensive care unit]—that's where it goes. It helped me feel like I could still be a mom in a way and be nurturing to somebody." The ritual of expressing the milk gave her some concrete action to aid in the grieving process via an activity she viewed as maternal. The baby's short life and her pain were not all for nothing. Her maternal identity was under threat, but she embodied motherhood still. And her milk carried it on.

Like pregnancy and childbirth, for many, producing breast milk fulfills a woman's destiny. Susan said that the hormone release from extended breastfeeding and pumping helped her cope with the stress of working motherhood. Rather than an added burden, milk production lubricated; it kept her system running smoothly and allowed her to be a good mother.

Susan was one of the few breastfeeders I talked to who thought it was particularly sad or unfortunate when a woman could not breastfeed, like she was missing out on an integral part of being a woman. We can read this sort of adamant belief that breastfeeding is part of the body's design in a couple of different ways. On the one hand, pigeonholing women as potential child-bearing breastfeeders can be a suffocating expectation. Women certainly experience full lives before they have children and if they never have children, before they breastfeed and if they never breastfeed. Men do not have to procreate to be seen as living up to their potential, and this should not be an expectation for women. But on the other hand, this seemingly biologically deterministic view that breastfeeding is by design can suggest that breastfeeding is a positive physiological experience with many advantages for the infant and for the breastfeeder. It is "natural" (an admittedly fraught concept), and it often works and feels good. None of these aspects of breastfeeding as a biological function need mean that the body *must* be used in this way, just that it should be embraced (and supported) as an option that can yield great results. Sex is like this too. It is supposedly an innate drive and a worthwhile pursuit for many (but not all), and the experience varies widely. Like the old joke about mediocre pizza, even when the experience is not optimal, it can still be good. Society needs to support the right to have sex however one wishes as long as it is not harming someone else. The same holds true for breastfeeding.

This discussion matters to breastfeeding because there are regulatory implications. When policy makers incorrectly reduce women to natural breastfeeders or when they assume breastfeeding to be a viable choice on par with formula, they harm the cause of procreative justice. The options to not breastfeed, or to breastfeed in exceptional ways, need to be respected even as we systematically remove the many structural and ideological barriers to breastfeeding.

The Mother Makes the Milk

An acquaintance told Harriet that "every drop of milk you give [your daughter] is 'liquid love.'" This advice helped her deal with the fear that supplementing with formula was a tier below breastfeeding in quality mothering. Each drop, imbued with the powerful metaphysical substance of love, purified the formula in the SNS. The mothers I spoke with, who virtually traveled to the ends of the earth to amass the ingredients for their lovingly homemade formulas, offered similar stories of transubstantiation.

"I can't call it formula!!" Kylie exclaimed doubly in an email. The raw cow's milk recipe she uses is "her milk," the "her" referring to Kylie's infant daughter. She writes, "She wasn't on the growth chart at 10 weeks of age and now she's at the 42%. Growth charts are overrated but you can see how much she's grown. . . . I LOVE HER MILK!" Kylie pumped what breast milk she could, and she nursed her daughter, but it was the not-formula that she made that caused her daughter to thrive. Sometimes it is the intent, the mother-love, that makes even formula into mother's milk.

The Milk Is Mothering

Providing breast milk is an act of mothering. It does not have to involve direct nursing. Exclusive pumpers know this. Some milk donors feel this way too. Many breastfeeders nurse their babies *and* provide pumped milk. Olivia said, "It was my parenting tool. It got them to sleep. It got them to sit still for five minutes. . . . It helped every 'owie.' When I stopped nursing, I lost all of my mothering. I didn't know what to do! And breast milk, you use it for earaches, for eye junk, for just whatever. It was the magic, magic cure for everything." For some, breastfeeding becomes central to their mothering. As with Olivia, learning other ways to nurture and calm children after weaning can be a jarring experience.

Valerie mothered her babies even when she was not present by providing them with her pumped milk: "I have always worked full-time. And so for me, giving my baby milk, even when I'm at work, that's the best thing that I can do when I am not with them. They can have my milk. . . . My milk is part of me, and so I still feel like I am very, very active in their care every day when I am pumping milk for them." Although she did not fetishize bonding at the breast, she did put herself into her milk. She was "very active in their care" even while her husband and the hired caregivers administered the bottles. The care put into pumping milk or mixing special formulas is a mothering activity not unlike cooking a family meal from scratch.

Aaliyah put herself into the milk too, and the stakes were a bit higher for her since she adopted her children: "I wasn't going to go through that bonded attachment process that pregnant women do. So I know it is beneficial for the baby even if they are not getting any milk, just the bond that is created. I know it is beneficial for the baby. But I think it was more so for me to help me with my healing process and to feel like I was really their mom. But I was actually able to give them a part of me even though I had not given birth to them." She appreciated the benefits of closeness and bonding that might occur even if there was no milk present in the breasts. The act of breastfeeding made her feel like a mother. Aaliyah did produce some milk, but even if she had not, there was that invisible "part of [her]" she mentioned that was getting transmitted through the breast. The love, the self, or the "feminine power" being passed along with breast milk is an intangible motivation for many breastfeeders. It can feel good to commit one's body completely to the project of mothering.

Being a parent at all is conventionally read as heteronormative in American society. And doing any of the physical work of a parent is always an embodied experience. Breastfeeding is an intensive version of this intimacy. And it becomes more wrapped up in gender than, say, dressing a child, merely because the culture defines breasts as feminine. This is not everyone's experience. Breasts and breastfeeding feel different depending on context and gender location. Some observers might criticize efforts to normalize queer breastfeeding as a type of mainstreaming: "Look at us, and see proof that gays are good parents too." But that is too simple an analysis. There are plenty of queer parents who breastfeed on their own terms. They want these practices to be accepted as "normal" as well.

But there are dangers in essentializing breast milk and bodies. These assumptions can be exclusionary, casting formula as the inferior option not just nutritionally but also spiritually. It can disrupt a woman's gender identity, making her feel less womanly if her body does not cooperate. Women may feel like they *must* breastfeed if physically capable, even when it does not work for their lives. In dystopian *Handmaid's Tale*–like imaginings, breastfeeding could become mandatory as a way to keep women in their place.

On the other hand, breast milk's special properties—if magical like this—can never be reproduced in a chemistry laboratory or packaged and sold on a shelf at a profit-making markup. The frequent scientific discoveries of breast milk's marvelous qualities only add to the mystery. Can it cure cancer, like some controversial research suggests?[14] Does it improve athletic performance and bodybuilding capabilities, as some people claim? There is strong observational evidence that breast milk helps infants in the NICU.[15] Breast milk has remarkable potential as research material, like surplus frozen embryos these days used for stem cell science.[16] If said research tells us definitively that breast milk kills cancer, it is hard to imagine putting the brakes on concerted and thorough efforts to commodify it. Maybe there is a protective advantage for breastfeeders' autonomy when it comes to their milk, at this moment, while breast milk remains relatively inscrutable.

There has yet to be a "white gold" rush, though there are reasons to fear that there will be.[17]

For now, elevating breast milk to "liquid love" puts it out of reach of soul-killing cyborgification. Contraptions like noisy pumps with all the parts and unwieldy SNS devices that require frequent cleaning lose some of their banality when juxtaposed with their part in the production and delivery of ambrosia suffused with maternal power. The medicalization and scientizing that distance breastfeeders from their bodies and their milk by scrutinizing the quantity and quality fade into the background. And what may have been a troublesome, inadequate body, with its leaking fluids, transforms into a temple of empowerment.

6 · FLUIDITY OF THE FAMILY
Making Kin

Here's to Oddkin—non-natalist and off-category! We must
find ways to celebrate low birth rates and personal, intimate
decisions to make flourishing and generous lives (including
innovating enduring kin—kinnovating) without making more
babies—urgently and especially, but not only, in wealthy high-
consumption and misery-exporting regions, nations, communities, families, and social classes.

—Donna J. Haraway in *Staying with the Trouble:*
Making Kin in the Chthulucene

Exceptional breastfeeding fosters "kinnovation." Haraway's
central concern in the book *Staying with the Trouble* is the earth's inability
to forever support humanity's exponential growth. Rather than narrow-
ing families, becoming smaller and more insular (and more demanding of
resources), she suggests expanding what family means, changing how we
"do family." Those innovators in the contemporary West who share milk, co-
nurse, induce lactation, wet-nurse, tandem nurse, or extend the number of
years they breastfeed are doing just that. They experience breastfeeding—in
all its diversity—as enhancing relatedness not just with their children but
with other breastfeeders with whom they may share milk or co-nurse.

This assumption of relatedness originates from society's long-held idea
that breast milk somehow contains the essence of a mother. (The science of
breast milk, which keeps showing that it is chock full of personalized, high-
quality compounds, does little to shift this perspective.) Sarah Franklin[1]

looks at how feminist anthropologists wrestle with "biological facts," which people use to naturalize restrictive gender roles in reproduction and to claim autonomous women's worlds. Men cannot have babies. Men cannot breastfeed. These truisms fall apart when we look closely at assisted reproductive technologies (as Franklin does) or at exceptional breastfeeding. In discussing in vitro fertilization, Franklin explains, "Reproductive substance is not automatically reproductive"; there have to be all sorts of social arrangements to make a baby. This pattern is also true for breastfeeding. We should not think of it as a "natural" part of raising children, without all the social relationships. The social relationships are what matter to the experience, not fulfilling some biological imperative.

Of course, all of these exceptional breastfeeding practices have been going on since antiquity,[2] and some groups have never stopped breastfeeding in ways that are now outside the medicalized mainstream. But there seems to be an emergent, progressive opportunity in exceptional breastfeeding— if it's not thoroughly regulated, medicalized, and commoditized—to reimagine and liberate the family. This reimagining needs to shift the dominant narrative if it is to impact policies. Our society as a whole can learn from those among us with historically less political power but with long experience in creative and expansive family building in the face of oppression—namely, black women, Native Americans, immigrants, Latinx communities, disabled parents, and queer families.

Off-category kin connected by breastfeeding and breast milk, on a scale of relatedness, may include casual kin, affective relations, oddkin (see Haraway 2016), and "other mothers" (see Collins 1990). The boundaries between these types of conceptual relatives can be blurry, and as always, they differ widely across social axes. Taken together, the types of kin created during breastfeeding add up to a more fluid notion of family.

CASUAL KIN

Kindred spirits in the breastfeeding world, variously understood as "sisterhood," "tribe," "culture," and "community," share affection and practical assistance.

Bailey had five children of her own when her sister suddenly passed away, leaving behind infant twins. She acquired all the milk they needed from donors she never met. One of the donors, trying to meet the demands of her own family, wrote about her inspiring, reciprocal connection with unknown recipients:

> I've been struggling all night with my own children. . . . I'm not proud to say that the devastation in Oklahoma only made me pause briefly. My messy house. The messes that my girls made earlier . . . has made me cringe every time. I have to go back into his bedroom to soothe one of them. My chores are not done. I am already behind from the messy, busy weekend. I am completely stressed out, and yet I had to find time to pump. I just bagged two days' worth of milk, and now I have to do it yet again. And I find myself again thinking about that mama and her baby, and I find myself thankful for my little milk buddies. I take my girls, their messes, and their neediness for granted. I need my little buddies for my reality check [emphasis added]. People think I am helping them. But I think maybe they are helping me.

She understands here that her "milk buddies"—a term of endearment that she invented—thrive on her milk and may suffer greatly without it. They reciprocate by needing her contribution. The relationship helped her put her own mundane stresses into perspective. While she could not muster what she considered an appropriate amount of empathy for the more distant "devastation in Oklahoma" (referring to some destructive tornadoes), she could do so for the "other mama and her baby." Those ties to other breastfeeding mothers are stronger for feeling more immediate. Bailey stayed connected with this donor and others on Facebook—she called them her "breast friends"—but mainly the relationship was in her heart and mind. She felt a kinship without having a face-to-face relationship.

Feelings of "kinship" may be fleeting and circumstantial. Some breastfeeders will nurse someone else's baby briefly at a La Leche League (LLL) meeting, for instance, just to pitch in or to help the infant learn to latch. Likely all of the breastfeeders in the room share similar hopes and goals for their infants. They do this for one another because they are members of a sisterhood. In her ethnography of anonymous egg donors and recipients, Monica Konrad finds that the gift-giving leads toward what she calls "irrelational kinship."[3] The eggs go "out there" to whomever—it is outside the control of the donor—and they are received from whomever—the recipients do not always get to choose the donor. But these nameless someones become kin of a sort. These deals involve genetic material, whereas milk can be reduced to a mere food. Still, both scenarios transfer some imagined relatedness along with the bodily substances. The ties are a bit more concrete than those of generic sisterhood with all women.

Black women, Latinas, and members of certain minority religious groups like Mormons and Muslims (in the United States) have a long history of communal mothering. In certain promaternal contexts, nobody bats an eyelash when others breastfeed a mother's baby or discipline someone else's child; everyone is already related, if distantly. A 2016 post on the Breastfeeding MAFIA's (Mothers Against Feeding Infants Artificially) Facebook page encouraged black women to breastfeed: "Surround yourself with people who have the same passion as you." The idea was to nurture an enduring community of like-minded mothers.

Many other breastfeeders have more self-contained, nuclear families and households. For them, "moms' groups," like the one I am still a part of (which grew out of a hospital-sponsored infant care support group), can pose a rare opportunity to establish significant new connections. "We would talk about these things and the challenges that we are facing and how [her new friend's] parents didn't get what we were doing. But we had each other," Tayshia recalled. She and her friends formed a neighborhood crunchy community of breastfeeding first-time mothers who were "trying some new ways and some old ways" of bringing up their children. In the absence of existing friends and family who "got it," they created out of whole cloth a replacement for extended, intergenerational family support.

Many new mothers report feeling a sense of removal from society.[4] When breastfeeders negotiate the stigma of their practices by avoiding going out in public or by holing themselves up in a private space in their own homes to nurse, the sense of isolation widens.[5] We tend to start our own small households (often moving far away from where we grow up in search of job opportunities), and we have to outsource so much of our childcare. Lacking "old wives" to impart wisdom, new parents who resist authorities' advice and directives in search of better or more "natural" ways are left to figure it out on their own. So-called moms' groups can fill this gap.

Some queer families, on the other hand, may have hard-won access to a nurturing community of mutual support. Marnie and her wife tried fertility treatments to get pregnant to no avail. One of their friends noticed that they no longer talked about it and asked them if they might be interested in adoption. The friend said, "Well, I have a friend of a friend who's a transguy who has an accidental pregnancy and is looking to place with a queer family. Can I pass along your information?" Marnie told me that four months later, she and her wife had a new baby.

These events exemplify the "strength of weak ties"[6] concept, in which networks intersect and individuals who do not know each other well provide key assistance like job leads or, in Marnie's case, a chance to adopt and become a mother. The queer community has developed its own support system for family building as a response to discrimination and is part of a broad project toward visibility, acceptance, and procreative justice.

Connie provided a story that illustrates the kinds of problems that can arise for lesbian and gender nonconforming parents who are trying to learn about breastfeeding:

> We were the only same-sex couple in the room, and so we did the whole class and [the instructor] talked about lactation and baby-led weaning. . . . She said, "All right, all mamas come with me into a separate room." Once we were in the room, she said, "Does your partner want to come?" I said—not knowing what we were to do—"She probably won't; let's leave her outside with the dads." I'm so grateful that she didn't. [The instructor] had some of the women squeeze their nipples to get some colostrum out, to show us how to get milk. And I felt uncomfortable because I felt all these other women are going to think I'm staring at them, so I didn't want to look too much. My partner is definitely more on the butch end of the spectrum, and I thought she would have died. She would've had absolute heart failure and been so embarrassed.

Though Connie and her wife worked hard to experience conception and pregnancy within a queer-friendly milieu—recall that they found *the* doctor for lesbians to work with—they still ended up confronting heteronormativity. The leader of the breastfeeding class showed up expecting moms- and dads-to-be with predictable concerns and conventional gender roles. For example, in order to conform to societal ideas about modesty, she separated the two groups: the breastfeeding "mamas" from the dads who had to wait outside. Of course, this unquestioned practice also reinforced gendered parenting roles, not leaving much room for another mother (or, for that matter, a father who might want to learn more about breastfeeding). The underlying concern seems to be that men or masculine-leaning lesbians might sexualize the women's breasts during the tutorial. In any case, Connie's partner narrowly escaped humiliation, but this close call underscores the necessity of queer-specific networks around family building.

The preexisting network under the queer umbrella has a few mechanisms for helping with breastfeeding such as how-to books geared toward queer families like Stephanie Brill's *The Essential Guide to Lesbian Conception, Pregnancy, and Birth*.[7] The internet is a particularly useful tool for connecting queer breastfeeding families,[8] but it is not enough to get information about how to induce lactation from online groups or books meant for parents via adoption or surrogacy. And it is not enough to hear from other lesbian or gay parents about the general tribulations of same-sex families. Queer breastfeeders want targeted support, and many get this from support groups that they find and form online.[9]

The "transguy" who birthed Marnie's baby breastfed before the placement and later provided pumped breast milk. He received emotional support and practical advice (like how to treat cracked nipples) from others on a private and "secret" transmasculine Facebook group where others respected his choices to give birth, to not parent, to breastfeed, and to continue to produce milk. These matters and his gender were not up for debate there. Fellow members of this queer internet community could focus instead on his actual immediate circumstances. His view of himself as a parent was limited. He gestated the baby and pitched in with some breast milk in the early months. But he enabled Marnie's queer parenthood. And by supporting Marnie's chosen infant feeding preference with his breast milk donations, theirs became an enduring relationship. This gestational parent's breast milk is a "donation" here because he did not share in the parenting. The milk that the baby got from Marnie's breast, however, cannot be categorized as a donation. The genetic tie matters much less than the social one in understanding the way milk and breastfeeding connect people.

Sometimes co-nursing and milk sharing with casual kin involves the whole family. For example, Eve's husband supported her pumping even though their baby died. Harriet modeled a community-minded ethic for her school-aged daughter, who called the pumped milk her mother shipped off "the milk for sick babies." And Jen's sister-in-law recruited her for ongoing donations to the sister-in-law's close friends.

For Kelly, milk sharing just made practical sense. She already deviated from a number of kinship norms in her roles as a co-nursing lesbian mom who adopted transracially. But the way she gave milk to an "internet acquaintance" with whom she shared mutual real-life friends seemed simultaneously old-fashioned and cutting edge. Kelly's story was not unusual among milk donors: she first got to know the other mother's needs by reading her blog, and then she offered the freezer stash, meeting her at a McDonald's parking lot with a cooler holding several gallons of pumped milk. They exchanged pleasantries and promptly went their separate ways. Susan Falls recognizes some local rules of "sociality" between breast milk donors and recipients in the American South, who socialize and "visit" with one another, frequently finding themselves in each other's homes, studiously avoiding the hot potato topics of religion and politics.[10]

This casual but friendly process differs from the highly monitored, regulated way that milk bank donations or blood donations get handled. And the breast milk parking lot drop is less legally precarious than at-home inseminations with a personal friend / sperm donor. Perhaps it is somewhat like buying a used car from a classified ad, except no money gets exchanged and there are no papers to file. It is neighborly—like giving away extra zucchini from one's garden—except milk donation is more than that too. We are unlikely to feel any cosmic or eternal connection to someone who sells us a car. But sharing milk—which, more than blood or sperm donation, comes from intensive bodily labor (pumping and sometimes special diets) by the donor—can establish more of an intimate, affective relationship, however brief. (At first glance, it seems that the implied intimacy or lack thereof works the same way for sperm donation. Just like with milk bank donations, when men sell their sperm to the sperm banks, they usually have no future relationship with the "recipient"[11] or any resulting children. Private arrangements vary widely, sometimes allowing ongoing intimate relationships in which men "help out" single women or lesbians who want to become mothers.)

Kelly donated her milk because, as she said, "I knew that there were babies out there that needed it and families that wanted it for their babies, and I worked really hard for that milk [laughing], and I didn't want it to go to waste." Upon discovering other would-be breastfeeders' stories—the abstract group of babies and families who are "out there"—faceless somebodies in need become more real. This often happens with correspondence—a getting-to-know-you phase, in which they may also check out each other's social media presence—and then may culminate in face-to-face interaction. That does not mean that peer donors and recipients become fast friends or family members. Deliberate pumping for a specific family engenders more of a relationship than donating to a milk bank or cleaning out a freezer of milk that is no longer needed. But in either case, a peculiar ally relationship may result. They are fellow accomplices in getting the babies fed outside institutional surveillance.

I do not want to suggest that there is more significance to this quasi kinship than there really is—many donors and recipients forget one another's names over time. Internet support groups have their limits. But the sisterhood (plus ties it creates) may function as a safeguard against regulatory intervention. To wit, the humor in these offbeat, off-script relationships is a sign of resistance. Respondents call their milk-sharing counterparts "bosom buddies" as well as "breast friends" and "the community chest." The nicknames make light of the taboo of sharing body fluids, the perpetual anxiety of biomedicine and public health. And the construction of these relationships as special resists the commodification that might turn what are now ad hoc activities into carefully managed and packaged market exchanges. Taking matters in hand and making them meaningful slows the progression toward tested, pasteurized, fortified breast milk bottled and arranged for sale on the supermarket shelf. Envisioning these connections as familial, locating milk sharing and instances of co-nursing within even a tenuous and temporary kinship network, keeps breastfeeding human and allows breastfeeders to retain some control over their bodies and their parenting.

AFFECTIVE RELATIONS

Not all milk sharing relationships are alike. Kerry donated her freezer stash to the local milk bank after her first child weaned. She contrasted this one-time event with her weekly milk donations to a friend. After both became pregnant around the same time, they went from being "acquaintance-y friends" to being close friends. "It started with, 'Hey, let's trade hand-me-downs,' and then she started to have milk supply problems again. I was like, 'Hey, I will give you milk too.'" Whereas casual kin do not have to ever actually meet in person to develop a vague sense of relatedness, affective relations like this one include milk-sharing or co-nursing breastfeeders who actually know each other and sustain their connection for at least the duration of the breastfeeding months or years. The length of time helps make the relationship a stronger one. I term these relations *affective* because they are emotional ties; the individuals are not genetically related, and they are not related through marriage. Instead they innovate a new relationship that differs from friendship. They become bonded not by blood but by milk.

Sometimes it is the response to a crisis or emergency that solidifies the relationship. By the time her friend received a breast cancer diagnosis, Sabine had birthed a second baby and was accustomed to sharing her milk and trading breastfeeding with a friend. The strength of this particular relationship came from its commitment; she pumped for months and made arrangements for a significant term of in-home breastfeeding care. Sabine planned to be a wet nurse and a proxy for her friend on a temporary, emergency basis.

Thomas and his husband received breast milk shipped by Mia, their gestational surrogate, for the first year of their baby's life. Though some surrogates perform this service as part of their contracts, others do so out of kindness—and, arguably, as a political action. Mia went to the trouble to pump and ship the milk as a continuation of living her beliefs about building families. Mia wants gay men to be able to be fathers together and enjoy parenthood. An experienced surrogate and mother herself, she shepherded them through the process beginning with fertilization. Mia convinced the couple that doing the insemination at home was preferable to—easier and more comfortable—than a clinical setting. During the pregnancy, they spoke daily and visited often. This contact slowly tapered off after the birth and dwindled even more after age one, when the baby no longer regularly received her milk. (She still shipped a little more in case the baby contracted a cold virus over the winter.) They never felt threatened by her or her relationship with the child. It eventually became unnecessary and impractical to communicate as often, though they kept "regular contact." Thomas said, "It is a really good relationship. A strong connection, just really from the beginning. It felt right. And it has felt right ever since. I have never questioned it." Mia will forever be known to the child as "a friend of the family" or as an "aunt." (They have yet to decide for sure.) The connection is a partial one—Thomas insists that Mia would never interfere in their "family dynamic"—but also a permanent one.

"Like family" networks can be just as integral to people's lives as more conventional family forms. My children have several "other brothers" who share a birth mother but were adopted by different parents. We get together for birthdays and holidays to help them connect with another. One family in particular has become part of our extended family, much like cousins. We do not share our daily lives, but our bonds are lasting. All the varieties of exceptional breastfeeding constitute nontraditional family building. And whereas the concept of "casual kin" puts milk sharing into the realm of human relationships that could be beyond the reach of authorities, affective relations borne of breastfeeding assistance are unforgettable. The relationships are deeper and more enduring.

ODDKIN

Rexi wanted to obtain her friends' and relatives' blessings and commitments to supporting her becoming a single parent. She invented a "generation ceremony," where she invited them to a Jewish-inflected ritual of her own devising. There are few social scripts available for a masculine-appearing, gender fluid person to enter parenthood alone and intentionally by insemination. She consulted an attorney, two rabbis, and a doctor friend in preparation. Serendipitously, Rexi ended up meeting her new partner, a transman, prior to giving birth, and they decided to give parenting a go. They planned to parent together, with Rexi doing the breastfeeding and her partner intimately involved in every other part of child rearing. Rexi "kinnovated" every step of the way. Rexi is not one for mainstreaming; she was not trying to fit into a particular gender role with her parenthood. The purpose of her innovative ritual ceremony was to anoint close friends and family as kin who would share in the work and joy of child rearing. Even without the new partner, who seemed game for unexpected parenthood, Rexi would not have embarked on parenthood all alone.

Tiana's version of kinnovating involved revitalizing and reclaiming African culture and African American motherhood. She explained that Oshun, an orisha (deity) in the West African Yoruba religion's pantheon, is said to "breastfeed all the babies." Tiana took inspiration from the songs, prayers, and "praise names" that honor Oshun as "the one that calms all of the babies when they are born, and so she does that through her song and also through her breast milk." Tiana, in sharing her breast milk, built on the long-standing tradition of black mothers' tight kinship networks. It is already common for black women to perform the mother role even if there is no "blood" relationship or legal guardianship. Like Oshun, Tiana would share her milk with "all the babies" if the opportunity presented itself.

Tiana and others told me that the community of black women in Atlanta who embrace alternative lifestyles and adhere to non-Christian religious traditions has started to formalize its connections. The community has milk-sharing collectives, mothering conferences, and midwifery apprenticeship programs that emphasize their common African roots and foster a greater breakdown of maternal boundaries within their community. Fellow mothers may feel uplifted and interconnected by nursing each other's babies or donating their milk to one another.

The Islamic kinship notion of "milk siblings" says that children nursed by the same woman become related (and therefore cannot be potential marriage partners). For Aaliyah's adoptive children, it sealed their sibling status. But if she or other black Muslim women were to co-nurse, they would be making new relatives outside Western society's conventional family unit.

Francine breastfed, in part, to establish equally close relationships with eleven of her children. She had fourteen in total: five adoptive and nine to whom she gave birth. She breastfed (all but the three she adopted as teenagers from West Africa) "because it is just common sense, doing something naturally. . . . We produce milk. Babies eat milk." In one sense, all she was doing was feeding her children the best way she could, just like she does around the family dinner table. Breastfeeding can be seen as simply another aspect of infant care like diapering or putting a baby down for a nap, though this was not Francine's primary view of it.

Like many breastfeeders, she focused on the bonding experience of breastfeeding: "There is just something special about being the only person who can feed your baby, and then when they are fussy, all they want is you." That special "something" puts breastfeeding in its own category apart from the other aspects of caregiving that another parent can do just as easily. Francine provided the nutrition, the connectedness, the warmth—every two hours in the early months. She committed herself to this effort for commonsense reasons and for spiritual reasons that strengthen kinship.

Francine contrasted the ease and joy of breastfeeding one of her adoptive children, who took to it "like a duck to water," over the "rough" experience she had nursing one of her birth children, suggesting that the connection started by pregnancy and birth does not necessarily determine the breastfeeding relationship. Rather, it was the breastfeeding that crystallized her identity and her experience as the mother. At one point, she suffered such exhaustion from tandem nursing that she was not thrilled about nursing the newest arrival. Yet she decided, "I didn't want to be like, 'Oh, yeah, I breastfed your brother, but not you.' So I decided to suck it up and do it again." Francine also felt like it was only fair to offer the same opportunity to each child; she became each infant's mother equally through the act of breastfeeding.

Oddkin in Haraway's vision likely includes all sorts of invented relatives, from long-term cohabitating, nonromantic friends to close adults who "adopt" one another for insurance purposes, to polyamorous families, to companion animals that spend their entire lives with us. Part of being human is having familial connections—one of the very few cultural universals—but how we define family varies drastically across cultures and eras. We do not always have agreed-upon categories, and when there is no specific language to describe our relationships, it becomes all too easy to dismiss their value. We risk not having legal protections. Conservative maneuvers to circumscribe what "family" can mean[12] are oppressive and, ultimately, bad for the earth. It is quite common for proponents of making marriage "only between a man and a woman" to insinuate that their aim is to protect the prospective children that originate from that union. With this distinctly natalist position, they assume that everyone wants to procreate but that only certain types of families are fit to do so.

Kin ties do not have to exclude children to qualify as "nonnatalist," however. Rexi had a child, but she surrounded herself and that child with kin whom she formally asked to help out. They become related to the child in this chosen family, and they did not need to participate in procreation to do so. Getting pregnant with sperm donation and being pregnant and birthing as a transmasculine person positions Rexi's parenthood as "off-category." Her exceptional breastfeeding is also off-category. Breastfeeding does not impact her gender, does not make her a mother, as I argued in the previous chapter. On the contrary, as breastfeeders actively resist essentialist characterizations, they help clear the path toward a wider variety of family forms.

Satisfying networks, like the one Tiana described, do not require men. (I talked with some mothers who set out to be single parents.) In this sort of world, grandmothers like Alice could relactate, freeing up young mothers to pursue their education or their careers. The point here is that Afrocentric communal breastfeeding and milk sharing may generate types of enduring oddkin that expand the family in ways old and new. For example, one black breastfeeder, Latisha, mused that she would have no problem nursing her sister's children because she was already "family," a sentiment that could transfer to a broader practice of family.

When foster and adoptive parents breastfeed the children joining their family, they experience a solidifying of the kinship bonds. There are both practical and ritual elements to establishing these ties between breastfeeder and child and between siblings. Whether they believe in the mystic powers of the fluid and that the milk connection is like a blood pact or they exalt emotional and spiritual "bonding," breastfeeding may ritually produce new kin. The phenomenon is not unlike the notion of "being married in the eyes of God" (by having intercourse) or being married in a religious ceremony versus being married by virtue of legal documents. The children are socially and legally recognized as theirs, but the breastfeeding adds that special "something" binds them together.

I do not mean to overstate exceptional breastfeeders' experience with or belief in the uncanny or transcendental origins of these kin ties (it's fair to be wary of ethnographers doing just that when writing about "exotic" cultures). Indeed, the breastfeeders I interviewed would be quick to highlight the decidedly practical reasons for their breastfeeding in exceptional ways. But with their off-category relationships, exceptional breastfeeders help free the family from constricting societal norms. Sharing in the breastfeeding makes it possible to innovate and to strengthen more varied kin connections.

OTHERMOTHERING

The useful term *othermothering*—all one word—was coined by Patricia Hill Collins,[13] sociologist and pioneer of black feminist thought. It refers to all the ways in which others besides the gestational "birth mother" take over or share the mothering duties and the mother role and relationship. In the following segment, I borrow this idea to consider how breastfeeding figures into the family building of comothers in same-sex marriages and partnerships. Co-nursing in this context is different from forging affective relations or even making oddkin. Othermothering with breastfeeding establishes

kinship with children and with one another. Sometimes co-nursing equal-
izes the mothers' relationship with the baby, and sometimes it does not.
Sometimes it brings the couple closer, and sometimes it does not.

Mommies and Me

"I absolutely feel closer to him that I would have been," declared Tara, who
induced lactation to co-nurse the son her wife birthed. Sandra, her wife,
encouraged Tara to induce lactation so that both could breastfeed their
coming baby; they would share the work more evenly and share in the
warm and fuzzy newborn bonding phase. Tara said of her wife, "She's super,
super excited that I'm feeding him. And super excited about my closeness
with him." As it happened, Tara came around to this way of thinking after
two and a half months of breastfeeding: "I feel really, really close with him,
and I feel like he relies on me and trusts me in a way that wouldn't be there
at this age. I was fully confident that that kind of trust and interdependence
would develop over time in the way that any kids develop that with their
nongestational parent over time, with their nonbreastfeeding parent. This
has accelerated that."

As Tara put it, it made "practical sense for [her] to try" inducing lactation and co-nursing, but it ended up being about more than getting the baby
healthy human milk. Achieving closeness with their son much earlier than
expected became central to her experience. Tara knew that time and attention would create a meaningful parent-child relationship just as it would
with any other nongestational parent. After all, many fathers, stepparents,
and adoptive mothers, to name a few common examples, enjoy close
relationships with their charges. Vice versa, plenty of birth parents prove
the corollary that giving birth or providing the gametes does not automatically make for a close familial bond with the child. The active performance
of *mothering*—again, a term that can apply to the care work done by a person of any gender identity—is likely to make the relationship authentic.[14]

Amelia said, "I'm not a very sort of maternal person" and "I really wanted
to minimize the ways in which I was going to have a sort of, like, 'mom' role
and Sami wasn't. I thought if she was to breastfeed too, then we would have
sort of that thing for her." Amelia, being the member of the couple with a
female reproductive system, expressed regret that she was "pushed into this
thing where it was definitely going to be me that was pregnant." She breastfed because "it is the right thing to do." But Amelia, who ended up "loving

it" after all, was keen to share the breastfeeding with her wife, who happened to be transfeminine. They already felt some satisfaction that their son "belongs to both of us now," as Amelia said, because after failed attempts with donor sperm, they ended up using gametes from each of them to conceive. But with breastfeeding, Sami could better embody the "mom role" too. (Remember that Sami does not equate mothering with femininity, and thus her breastfeeding is less of a gender story. For her, mothering is all about the relationship with the child.)

Co-nursing can begin as a mechanism for solidifying what are seen as biological ties. Jeri, whose egg was implanted into the uterus of her partner, said, "I wanted to [breastfeed] because, one, I am genetically connected to her, and I just thought it would be amazing to have that genetic connection and closeness, and the ability to bond with her in that way is something that, I mean, I couldn't believe that I would have the opportunity to do it. So even though it was a lot of work, it was totally worth it to be able to."

Genetic connections matter to families in varying degrees.[15] Some queer parents (and adoptive parents and stepparents) view genetic ties as irrelevant or, perhaps like Sami and Amelia, as a bonus. To be sure, genetic connections provide some legal standing when rights and responsibilities come under contention in court or in medical contexts. Queer families feel this ever-looming external threat to their families' integrity. Yet arguably, what was "amazing" about Jeri breastfeeding was the opportunity for the closeness. In our interview, she often returned to this benefit; she and her baby shared an intimate attachment that Jeri attributed to breastfeeding. Her early interest in breastfeeding as a way to continue her solely *biological* relationship with the baby faded into the background. Instead she discovered that the strength of their *kin* relationship came from the intimacy of breastfeeding and other daily mothering practices.

For comothers Aurora and Beth Ann, "There was never really any question. As soon as we found out it was possible, it was this thing that was going to happen. We're all about breastfeeding," said Aurora. (Beth Ann cut it in to agree.) Beth Ann, the mother who induced lactation, added, "A lot of people have asked about [Aurora's] jealousy and how we share it and everything. We never even realized that those negative emotions could be involved. There was no jealousy." Instead, these two, like several of the other co-nursing couples I spoke with, saw only benefits to the arrangement. As Tara did, the parents welcomed the practical assistance but emphasized the meaningful relationship-building. Aurora said, "They have the sweetest relationship. And I've seen a lot of partners who—I mean, it is hard for them to always have to give the baby to the breastfeeding mother. . . . They feel just useless that they have to give the baby back. I love it that she gets to share that too. I think it is such a sweet connection. Obviously they have an amazing bond. They would even if she wasn't breastfeeding, but she spends a lot of time with her breastfeeding." Aurora realized that unlike other breastfeeding mothers, she could take a shower whenever she wanted, get comparatively more sleep, and leave the house to run errands even during those early months when their baby seemed to be nursing constantly.

Kelly, a co-nursing lesbian comother, contrasted her experiences with breastfeeding and bottle-feeding:

> It's built-in snuggling. Especially in the middle of the night with the baby, who was not sleeping through the night ever, just being able to roll over and nurse him and not have to get out of bed was worth a lot. We've done both. We had foster babies, and we got up every two hours making a bottle and having the baby in the other room in a crib. It's just a completely different kind of parenting. I love my foster daughter, and I would not say that my bond with her was any less than my bond with my son, but it was definitely a totally different kind of parenting, and I definitely prefer being able to lay on my ass than get up and make a bottle. [Laughs]

Though the "amazing bond" was the actual selling point for Aurora and Beth Ann, none of these mothers thought they had some special lock on closeness just because they were breastfeeding. They did not suggest that bottle-feeding parents or the nonbreastfeeders in the family lacked the same kinds of meaningful connections with their babies. Instead, they experienced breastfeeding as "built-in snuggling" (to borrow from Kelly's description) that catalyzed their bonding.

This "different kind of parenting" theme that Kelly mentioned offers multiple insights. She made the observation that breastfeeding is the easier, "lazier" of the two options. Indeed, *breastsleeping*, the term coined by anthropologists James McKenna and Lee Gettler,[16] connotes the seamless (if fitful) integration of sleep and breastfeeding among breastfeeders who "bedshare" with their nurslings. The researchers and breastfeeders in this study tend to agree that this practice fosters attachment.[17]

For Kelly, the parenting difference between breastsleeping and getting up to make bottles just made for disparate bonding opportunities; she loved all of her babies. With bottle-feeding, the parent may have to put forth more effort—like getting up and then cradling and rocking the baby, making eye contact, perhaps going skin-to-skin, and singing and shushing—but there is love in that effort. Exclusive pumpers do all of this plus frequent pumping and milk management. Also recall that some study participants, such as Lanie whose school-aged son did shirtless "on-sies" and gay father Thomas who offered breast milk in a bottle to his infant skin-to-skin, considered their practices to be variations on breastfeeding. In any case, as with breastsleeping, the mothering that goes along with bottle-feeding shapes the relationship and feeds back into the affection and mutual attachment. Many fathers and others provide infant care and support the breastfeeder by sometimes giving bottles of pumped milk or formula. These intimate moments also make for parent-child attachment.

Othermothering with breastfeeding can minimize the differences in "maternal identity" when one parent gave birth and the other did not.[18] Other times, negotiating breastfeeding can be fraught. For Joanie, the prospect of co-nursing was an "emotional landmine." She said, "[My wife] also really wanted to try to breastfeed our second child, so she took domperidone and tried to do that, but I think it was a bit of a point of contention between us because I did not try to do that with [our first child]. And I kind of wanted to own that. With [the second child]." Joanie wanted exclusive ownership rights between herself and her daughter, and she achieved this first by gestation and birth and later by breastfeeding. She felt OK about not breastfeeding her son, their first child, because her wife took the first turn in having that sort of relationship and because Joanie's brother provided the sperm for that pregnancy. She shared a genetic tie, so she could virtually tick off the box that proved her relatedness.

Joanie went on to explain that her wife wanted to breastfeed to establish *her* relatedness, "Since my ex was unrelated to her daughter, and I was related to her son, she felt like she wanted to [breastfeed] anyway to deepen her relationship with her. You know, deepen that initial bond." The couple fought over this, and the partner ended up being unable to adequately induce lactation anyway. Although as a lesbian couple they subverted norms about who should be parents in the first place, Joanie applied other norms to her narratives of relatedness. She called up genetic and biologistic assumptions about making kin. For Joanie, sharing genes (through her brother's sperm donation) solidified her relationship with the first child. But she seemed to assume that her partner must have a stronger bond because she was the only one to breastfeed that infant.

In this way of thinking, just holding and a feeding a baby without actually breastfeeding cannot produce the same "deep" relationship as breastfeeding. Would the connection be deeper for Joanie's partner because the breastfeeder herself experienced pleasurable sensations and/or because of the physiological (and metaphysical) feedback between breastfeeder and nursling? Would Joanie's partner be more related to the baby because milk is a bodily substance she could share like the brother shared his sperm? All of these ideas are in play, though they remain internally inconsistent. This apparent intimate jealousy happens against a backdrop of shaky social and legal standing as lesbian comothers in a heteronormative society. For them, relatedness is at risk, and it is a source of confusion.

Comother Love

As Marnie explained, breastfeeding offers benefits that she did not want to give up even though her "jealous" partner disapproved. Marnie, her partner reportedly feared, could end up having a closer relationship to their adoptive child, leaving the partner frozen out of the family in a way:

> So you know it is just like this weird devaluation of what I am doing from my very kind of butch trans partner, and it is really messing with my head. Like I constantly talk about it in therapy. It is all I talk about because I am just so pissed off. My partner said the other night, "So the baby is having his four month sleep regression," which he thinks is great fun, but I really miss sleep. I said to my partner, "So I nursed him the other night," and my partner went off the deep end about it and was like, "I do not know why you think it comforts him, it probably just comforts you."

Marnie's partner thought that the amount of nutrition Marnie could offer was negligible, so breastfeeding did not make sense. Comfort nursing for the baby's sake did not figure into her partner's understanding. But Marnie, who conceded that the benefits were mutual between her and the baby, insisted that it is the partner's discomfort with the prospect of breastfeeding (as a transman) at the root of their conflict: "I was like, 'Really dude, you are going to go there? Why don't you come and have him suck on your nipple for five minutes and see how that feels?'" She also pointedly argued that, technically, her partner could breastfeed too. Marnie knew these were fighting words. But her partner's gender experience and apparent jealousy seemed to be getting in the way of Marnie's freedom to breastfeed. Marnie said, "It is part of the hallmark of our couplehood that we bicker, but having a baby has really messed with our gender roles . . . which has made things a little tedious."

Breastfeeding is almost destined to fail when it becomes a point of contention. Virtually every breastfeeder and every lactation professional I talked to emphasized "support" as the primary factor in breastfeeding success. Support can come from many directions, from medical service providers to hospital policies to friends and family.[19] Emotional and practical support, or lack thereof, in a breastfeeder's primary relationship likely makes or breaks the experience. The emotional toll on Marnie, who found herself having to sneak around to breastfeed in secret, contributed to the dwindling of her milk supply. She nursed less often, which diminished production, and the stress of the situation may have impacted her capacity to produce milk. She felt sabotaged by her partner. The relationship suffered. While Marnie thought the two could patch things up, the bitterness about breastfeeding was particularly difficult for her to get past.

Obviously, each comothering relationship is different. Connie checked in with her wife about breastfeeding, "I came home and I said to her, 'I feel bad because I've never asked you, but would you ever have any interest in breastfeeding? And I think her response was, 'Oh, hell no!' [Laughing]." Connie mentioned that her wife has a more butch identity and that the mere prospect of pregnancy, childbirth, and breastfeeding is funny because "those things just don't occur to her."

But Connie's wife stayed intimately involved in the breastfeeding relationship. "The milk is in! The milk is in!" she enthused in the middle of the night when she realized that Connie's breasts were engorged a few days postbirth. Connie made it clear that her wife's participation was complete even though the baby only suckled on Connie's breasts: "[My wife] wakes up for almost every single middle-of-the-night feed. She will take him, when I am done nursing on one side . . . and she will burp him and give him back to me. She's been great." Breastfeeding, then, did not divide the couple; it united them.

For some comothers, shared breastfeeding improves their relationship. And this improvement can happen because they lighten one another's workload and because it becomes an intimate project that they embark on together. Kris and Rachel set out to co-nurse with limited expectations, as Kris explained:

> Rachel and I always just both wanted to breastfeed, but we didn't really know very much about it. In both our first pregnancies, we thought, "Well, this is something we're going to try, and we'll give it six months and see how it's going." . . . Rachel is extraordinarily sensitive, so she was concerned about the physical aspect of nursing and whether that would be very uncomfortable for her. I have, it's a little hard to tell in maternity clothes . . . a pretty masculine gender orientation, and so for me, being sort of in touch with that part of my body, enjoying this very feminine thing, especially in public, was very intimidating.

Kris accepted the gender contrast rather than continuing to experience her breasts as disembodied and not truly part of her. Realizing first that she would have to get "in touch with that part of [her] body," Kris eventually breastfed so much as to feel very comfortable doing so anywhere. Both mothers breastfed for a couple of years despite their initial worries. As a consequence, "He's really attached to both of us. I would say he's equally attached to both of us," said Kris. "Oh, yeah. For sure," affirmed Rachel. Whereas Marnie's partner worried about unequal attachment when only one parent breastfed, Rachel and Kris (as well as other co-nursing lesbian couples I talked with) cherished this equality not only as a way to provide their child with maximum love but also as a way to improve (even to repair) their relationship with one another and to strengthen the family overall. Kris said, "I think [our son] is a really, a really joyful, present, nonanxious creature, which I think makes me feel good for [breastfeeding] the last couple years. Yeah, I would say Rachel and I are very much on the same page in terms of our parenting, which has been a real boon for us because for any interpersonal struggles that we have worked through in our marriage, parenting has just never—we've always been on the same page about it."

Co-nursing made mothering easier, and it was a "boon" to them for this reason and because it was an area of strong agreement and family cooperation. Breastfeeding was not the only aspect of their self-described "holistic" approach to parenting—they also shared approaches to cosleeping, diet, and discipline—but it was one of the primary ways in which they committed to being a family (the other ways included taking turns with insemination and pregnancy: "two wombs, no waiting!" Rachel joked).

Exceptional breastfeeders who share milk and nursing innovate and strengthen kinship with these efforts. Novel types of relationships emerge, but this new path can be meandering and bumpy. Mainstream assumptions about gender and kinship can translate into interpersonal conflict as well as limiting social policies. Many of the exceptional breastfeeders I interviewed pushed back to reach their goals, expanding their kin relationships as a result. They focused on the immediate needs of their own families. As they discovered satisfaction and negotiated unreasonable barriers along their journeys with exceptional breastfeeding, many of these parents wished to spread the good word on lessons learned. It's an after-the-fact story. Through their trials with breastfeeding, they stumble onto something new that offers liberation. In the next chapter, I trace the ways in which exceptional breastfeeders reach out beyond their own families and close communities to forge solidarity with all sorts of parents.

7 · "OUTPOURING OF SUPPORT"
Embodied Solidarity

My friends don't sell [their milk]. They do milk sharing for
the love.
                                                        —Winnie

Social movements are inherently hopeful things.
        —Barbara Katz Rothman, *A Bun in the Oven:*
How the Food and Birth Movements Resist Industrialization

Exceptional breastfeeders need each other. They find one
another online, at La Leche League (LLL) meetings, in breastfeeding
classes offered by hospitals, at birth centers, through midwifery collectives,
and within their extended social networks. In talking with them, I was struck
by their shared, abiding impulse to provide support to other parents without regard to others' social politics and parenting choices. Donna captured
the common sentiment: "Try your best, and whatever happens, happens; it
doesn't matter how you end up feeding your baby. Just that you love your
baby." Exceptional breastfeeders, having suffered sanctimonious treatment
by others, understand that the choices they and others make never occur in
a vacuum. They physically support one another outside of the oppressive
mommy wars discourses and without regard to institutional boundaries
(like regulating milk sharing). Together, with a sort of embodied solidarity,
exceptional breastfeeders resist biomedicine and other authorities that
might impede their breastfeeding goals. Ethnographer Susan Falls describes

a diffuse *communitas*, or emotion-heavy togetherness, among the milk sharers she studied, many of whom extend themselves outside of their usual
political and religious circles.[1] The exceptional breastfeeders I interviewed
build this solidarity using several mechanisms that I delineate here into
four interlocking themes: inspiration-seeking, networking, perspective-
taking, and reciprocity. Exceptional breastfeeders are only human, of
course, and none of this is to suggest that they are a special class immune
to ethnocentrism. Their relative privileges always influence their experiences, but nevertheless, they share a distinct recognition that their way
of parenting cannot possibly be the only morally correct way to do it. Many
exceptional breastfeeders wind up passionate not just about breastfeeding
but about breastfeeding justice. I like Susan Falls's adventurous suggestion
that lactivists call themselves *galactivists* (the word *galaxy* originates from
gala—meaning "milk"—in ancient Greek) to indicate a more universal and
inclusive approach to breastfeeding advocacy.[2]

INSPIRATION-SEEKING

Exceptional breastfeeders cull lessons from others' stories to feel better about themselves and to learn of creative ways of breastfeeding. For
example, Eve talked about her experience with donating her milk when her
baby passed away in order to let other grieving mothers know that it is an
option. Her story can also inspire *anyone* who wants to donate or who seeks
a reason to keep going with breastfeeding.

Breastfeeders may look to others in order to normalize their own circumstances. "Oh, my breasts aren't weird," realized Sabine after attending LLL
meetings and hanging around with attachment parenting groups, wherein
breastfeeders routinely nursed uncovered. "When you see any woman
topless in a[n] R-rated movie, in print, they're always little and perky," she
explained. Seeing other woman helped her conclude that her large areolas
were nothing to be ashamed of and made her less self-conscious about nursing in public.

Exceptional breastfeeders in particular will both seek out and share
their own breastfeeding life hacks and motivations. Tayshia, for instance,
read "a lot of stories: women's stories, mama stories," over a period of about
six months before she attempted to wean her daughter—which she finally

did when the girl reached age four. And Roxanne started a blog, initially to explain her seemingly quirky procreative choices to skeptical family members, but it grew into a popular stop on the internet for would-be exceptional breastfeeders seeking advice and inspiration. After having exclusively breastfed for five months, one black woman posted an announcement to that effect on a public breastfeeding site online. She wrote in all caps, "LOOK AT ME NOW." Her post included a story of how others bashed her for breastfeeding by saying things like, "Get that baby some real milk," "Don't ask me to babysit because I'll get that baby a can of formula," and "Oh, you think you white?" She followed this with a list of the healthful benefits of breastfeeding. Not only was she proud of surviving these negative interactions and continuing to breastfeed, but she wanted others to feel inspired to do the same. She wrote, "This page gives me the strength I need to keep going. . . . Every time I wanted to quit, I see someone on this page fighting through the same thing I'm going through, and that's all the support I need." A study from 1993 that asked "Does breastfeeding empower women?" found that low-income minority women described "telling the world" as a component of their empowerment.[3]

Some go online to get specific supports for unusual circumstances. Sheena noticed, "There is a stigma . . . around donor milk," which she deemed to be "weird." A leitmotif of "weirdness" pervades the interviews; there is much narrative work and emotion around the unfamiliar and taboo aspects of exceptional breastfeeding. One way to cope with the strangeness and the stigma of exceptional breastfeeding is to talk about it and perhaps to laugh at the funny situations it brings about. Another key mitigation strategy is to find and befriend kindred souls. To this end, Sheena joined a Facebook group called Mommy2Mommy, composed of mothers in her own geographic community, several of whom she got to know in person. The site helped her locate "lots of moms who need milk," and she no longer felt isolated in her breastfeeding difficulties. The group was far from a perfect respite from motherhood controversies, though. Sheena noted a couple of its limitations: mothers, she worried, may have sought medical advice there instead of taking their children to the doctor promptly, and certain topics—like vaccination—were always explosive. Still, she could see herself in others' milk supply struggles and conclude that her experience was within the range of common experiences and not so pathological.

Sometimes online groups—be they large public forums or small local groups made up of real-life friends—feel like the place to turn when breast-feeding seems to be going horribly awry. One particular post, made at eleven minutes past midnight on a lactation consultant's Facebook page (which the users allowed me to observe), is absolutely typical: "I don't want to go to formula, but I've barely had any sleep for days and I'm losing my mind. Please someone help with tips or advice. Maybe a few encouraging words. I'm trying so hard not to breakdown."[4] This first-time mother's immediate family members lacked the experience to help, and the lactation consultant was unavailable at that hour. But the virtual community had her back, and she knew how to ask for what she needed from them. As expected, others who were up at that hour rushed to soothe her worries about her milk not having come in yet a few days postbirth. They related their own nail-biting tales of having waited for the milk for what seemed an interminable three, four, even seven days.

It is worth noting that a post on the same site that included the question "When did you know breastfeeding wasn't going to work for you?" elicited the same kind of support for that worried mother too. In their responses, the commenters gave accounts of their own trials, some finding their way to months of relatively trouble-free breastfeeding, others coming to terms with the bottle-feeding option and learning to appreciate its advantages.

These communities offer inspiration, tips, and solace, usually without prejudice. There is trollish behavior, of course. Particularly on the larger sites, so-called sanctimommies, hiding behind a false sense of anonymity, may cast judgment. A few instigators may offer unhelpful comments like, "You have to allow your child to grow appropriately. Feeding them on the tittie [sic] at four is stagnation." Occasionally, others' choices induce rage. When one breastfeeding site featured a story on Transgender Remembrance Day about Trevor MacDonald, a transman and LLL leader, most commenters marveled at his dedication; I tallied "awesome" as the most frequent response from the scores of posts. But a few commenters ranted about gender rules and even resorted to name-calling and deliberate gender misidentification (e.g., "That is wretched. . . . He can't breastfeed—let's call it [sic] what it truly is, a woman"). But thankfully, there are mechanisms in place to create judgment-free zones, including group moderators who delete troublesome posts; keep groups invitation-only, private, and/or "secret"; censure and contradict mean-spirited or narrow-minded commenters, and post rules of conduct and reminders of those rules. The sheer number of options these days makes it possible to steer clear of sites that fail to keep the hurtful comments at bay. Exceptional breastfeeders, whatever their path, can usually find comfortable niches on the internet, they told me.

More so than in person, the internet allows for communities to arise around narrow interests and very specific circumstances. After searching for answers for months from doctors, from books, from lactation consultants, and from LLL groups, Amy discovered a Facebook forum in which others like her offered practical advice for continuing to breastfeed despite having insufficient glandular tissue (IGT): "[It] actually has, I don't know, one thousand or so members who all have this, basically IGT or something, where no matter how much you try to nurse, your supply is never a full supply. So you do the things like cofeeding, the SNS [supplemental nursing system], donor milk; you try to make up for it to feed your baby." Amy talked about these various options almost as if they were normative—"you do the things"—because, together, these exceptional breastfeeders—not medical authorities—constructed a protocol where there was no norm. Beyond the emotional support and commiserating, there are doable solutions. As they figure things out, these exceptional breastfeeders are blazing a trail for others.

Sometimes just seeing what others can do can make all the difference. Sabine, by then an experienced breastfeeder, attended LLL meetings mainly to offer support:

> The people who come to La Leche League meetings are in the thick of what I went through with my son for the first three to six months. They're dealing with bad latch; they're dealing with tongue-tie;[5] they're dealing with a baby that screams at the breast; they're dealing with under- or oversupply. I think that it's beneficial for someone to be there who can say, "I've been there. It sucks; it's hard—it'll get better. You can stick it out. It can be OK; you can keep this nursing relationship going." [Laughs] And also just to say, "You're not alone there." Because, like I said, all the images are of these Madonna-nursing-the-baby kinds of peaceful, beautiful images, and it doesn't always look like that.

Thanks to her experiential knowledge of breastfeeding, having dealt with the standard stumbling blocks, Sabine was in a position to inspire others. She was not there for the camaraderie. Instead, Sabine assumed the role of an accidental activist, embracing breastfeeding advocacy and encouraging others to keep trying. The LLL meeting (as well as other breastfeeding support groups) can be more realistic than the "inspiring images" of soft-focus portraits of a mother and baby breastfeeding that Lily noticed on the wall of her local Women, Infants, and Children Food and Nutrition Service (WIC) office. A room full of breastfeeders featured screaming babies, latch problems, and "nervous" and "stressed" parents—as Sabine noted—who were far from photo-ready. Such a room may also provide glimpses of tandem nursing, breastfeeding toddlers or even preschoolers, cofeeding, and the use of supplementers. (Some LLL groups support mixed feeding and pumping, and others do not. Participants who cannot comply with the doctrines sometimes feel negatively judged and stop attending.) By seeing the many ways breastfeeding can look and the various ways it can be accomplished, more breastfeeders can persevere. They may be less apt to think that their particular issues are out of bounds and more likely to grasp that there is a sizeable learning curve for almost everyone.

Vanessa did not know that anyone would or could relactate and breastfeed a child who was not "very young" until she came across a 1993 La Leche article titled, "Nursing Julia: My Supreme Challenge," by Darillyn Starr. This heartfelt story gave her the courage to try it, with extremely positive results for her traumatized adoptive daughter. Vanessa went on to share *her* story with others—like me—because she knew from experience the power of just finding out what is possible.

Mira was also spurred to action when she noticed a way to help: "I was just about to have my fourth [child], and I saw that all of these women were complaining about how hard it is to use the supplementer. I was like, 'No, it's not! Let me show you.' And I did this video. I was like, 'Look here, you clean it like this. You don't use any of those materials; it is so much easier. And then you flip it on. Just so much easier. If you could just come to my house, I will just show you.'" Mira understood that reaching out like this really could mean the difference between someone continuing to nurse or stopping in frustration.

Emie, a lactation consultant, put it this way: "That 'keep trying, honey' method of breastfeeding support doesn't work." Practical support—

metaphorically taking the other breastfeeder by the hand—and showing them what to do can be more effective. There is much to be said for the bodily part of "embodied solidarity." These kinds of supports are not clinical but generously personal.

Liza, who lives in a rural area, serendipitously discovered her proximity to another breastfeeder of a child who was adopted. This woman showed Liza the ropes—or "tubes," as it were—in using the Lact-Aid supplementer. This pattern represents a nascent grassroots movement that is becoming exponentially more common—or at least more commonly known. Some breastfeeders I talked to recalled finding milk donors and recipients on what are now old-fashioned message boards and LISTSERVs, even classified ads. In 2008, when my second son was a newborn, it was still quite unusual to share milk online. The options are plentiful now, and these sorts of transactions happen every day. Just by logging into breastfeeding-related sites and forums, visitors can read others' online milk-sharing interactions and observe discussions about other kinds of exceptional breastfeeding. This exposure inspires some caregivers to try alternate routes to breastfeeding.

Exceptional breastfeeders seeking inspiration sometimes have to take the bad along with the good. Dorinne lamented that her group of "special feeders"—breastfeeders using a supplementer "for one reason or another"—who used to meet at a church, recently disbanded and moved to an online format. In some ways, the change was for the better: "They would have to get up and get dressed and get the kids there and get into the church. We can't necessarily wait two weeks to get our questions answered or meet another mom who is going through the same thing they are." But in another way, as Dorinne said, "[It is] kind of sad. Kind of strange. A sign of the times that a Facebook page takes the place of moms meeting in person."

Exceptional breastfeeders negotiate their online experience with varying degrees of aplomb to get a diversity of needs met. Latisha spent time on two sites specifically for "black moms." There she found "support, information that I had no idea about before breastfeeding. The different things you can use breast milk for and the different natural remedies, like when you encounter a breast issue, an infection, or cracking of the nipples. Just more holistic, natural things. I don't want to expose my baby to unnecessary chemicals." This information was both practical and affirming of her choices to breastfeed and to mother "naturally," in contrast to commercial interests. One of the two groups, Black Women Do Breastfeed (BWDBF), whose name is at once a defense and an inspirational statement, provided more options that Latisha had "no idea about." This information is not integrated into clinical protocols, and it is no longer installed in family memory. But it can be found in these special communities online and in person.

Marnie expanded her network when she butted up against the limits of what her more familiar community had to offer: "[Getting support from LLL groups] is kind of screwy because, at least the people I know in New York who belong to them, are these like relatively liberal, left-wing, feminist radicals. I just feel like there is a disjoint there. I also find them pretty militant in how they talk about breastfeeding. We share nothing in common, I really have to say."

Even though they are Marnie's "people" politically and socially, their breastfeeding narrow-mindedness pushed her away. Their unexamined, able-bodied privilege in being able to provide sufficient breast milk on demand allowed them to pooh-pooh bottles and formula as less natural, less organic, less self-actualized choices that support capitalism and contribute to environmental degradation. They may not follow the old guard LLL party line about staying at home and fulfilling their supposedly intended role as mothers, but these ersatz feminists seem to take the breastfeeding part of the doctrine for granted. In search of understanding, Marnie fled into the virtual arms of what seemed to her to be some very unexpected comrades:

> It is really bizarre because lots of them are just creepy Christian—God called them to adopt, and they are going to save some babies from the Congo and crazy shit. But in kind of a broader way, they are the people that most get what I am going through in terms of having a baby that is not biologically or genetically related to me. And also in thinking about different types of nourishment and feeding. There is a great adoptive breastfeeding community on Facebook, and then I belong to The Bump message board. I don't even know what media corporation owns it, but it is somehow connected to Pampers. And those women have a spin-off group on Facebook. So I spend a lot of time there.

At one intersection, Marnie was an adoptive breastfeeder who sought support and advice from others who "get it." But her same-sex partnership is what led her to adoption, not any kind of savior complex. Indeed, the conservative politics and religion behind some folks' rationale for adoption—as opposition to abortion or as rescuing children from a life of poverty—chafe against Marnie's beliefs and identity. As a lefty and a lesbian, Marnie found these other breastfeeders to be "bizarre" and "creepy," trafficking in "crazy shit." And yet her immediate needs as an exceptional breastfeeder continued to bring her into contact with them. She discovered that she had to look in one direction for support for her queer family building and another for support for her queer—as in nonnormative—breastfeeding strategy (inducing lactation and using an SNS). There are bridges being built here, though.

NETWORKING

"I think it is important now to help other moms. One of my very, very good friends and neighbor has a son who is five months younger than my son and has a huge oversupply. I have introduced her to breast milk sharing," said Donna, who once had to deal with low supply herself. She became wistful as she thought about what a great resource this friend could have been back when Donna needed milk. Later, she was "just trying to use the experience to help other moms." This pattern of encountering and then solving difficulties with one's own breastfeeding and then later trying to connect others, whether the basis is milk sharing or advice giving, leads some exceptional breastfeeders to embrace a politics of liberating breastfeeding. They are not just helping out a friend or acquiring help for themselves anymore but actively intervening, putting third parties together to promote exceptional breastfeeding. These embracers sell the idea to others that they too can make breastfeeding work as long as they have the right connections. And these original exceptional breastfeeders establish those networks for others' use.

Like Donna, Kadijah never set out to broker milk. But when she began working as a home birth doula, it came with the territory—though it was not something she got paid to do. In one case, Kadijah got to know a birthing surrogate and arranged for the surrogate to pump her milk for donation to a pair of adoptive fathers. Kadijah said proudly, "After giving birth to the baby that she was carrying for another family, she pumped." Kadijah became a hub in a network of families helping other families. And in her circles, these were all black families, which was a significant detail given the attitude among the previous generation of black mothers: "You don't [breastfeed]. . . . It was just something you didn't talk about."

It is easy to feel rejected when one's milk is, well, rejected. When Susan, an exclusive pumper, decided it was time to pump extra milk to help other breastfeeders who were having low supply troubles, she discovered that having taken fenugreek to increase her milk supply put her in the "no, thank you" category by the local milk bank. Their policies shut her out. Susan wrote in an email, "I kinda started to feel like I was doing all this work, and no one wanted my milk! I actually vented about it to my [exclusive pumping] Facebook support group. Of course, they assured me that my milk was still valuable and there were actually a few women who hoped I would be willing to ship it to them (with them reimbursing shipping costs)." The online community gave her that nudge she sought to keep going in the face of bureaucratic dismissal and inconsiderate peers. Her online plea for commiseration in turn led to instant networking. Often, real-life connections happen, and inspiration-seeking goes hand in hand with networking.

One breastfeeding support group that I observed in person and online arranged get-togethers around town. The members provided each other with advice about where in the area to buy certain low-flow bottle nipples (ones that are better to help babies continue to breastfeed) and met up to share pump parts and other baby gear. They also shared secrets online in their closed Facebook group about how to acquire the drug domperidone from overseas in ways that fool U.S. Customs. In person, I saw these breastfeeders share the tricks of domperidone acquisition with conspiratorial giggles and sardonic smiles. Technically, I suppose, they were conspiring to break the law by getting the domperidone illegally, but it was not a "crime" for which they were likely to be called to account. They bonded over this minor breach in pursuit of the same goal: breastfeeding success. They were practicing good intimate citizenship within a resistance culture. The general public may disapprove of their rule breaking, but among "good mothers" just trying to breastfeed as prescribed, this practice was morally correct. Just as Jennifer Reich observed of well-off mothers who reject vaccines, they see themselves as "independent, thoughtful, and deliberate."[6]

These support networks may arise organically or may be part of a more organized community like LLL or a preexisting online forum. At the same time that struggling breastfeeders find inspiration and practical help within these networks, their praxis—embodying exceptional breastfeeding—opens up new perspectives on how nurturing and nourishment can look.

PERSPECTIVE-TAKING

> I'm not trying to belittle anybody who chooses to bottle-feed. I think whatever way you can take care of your kids is OK for you.
>
> —Jen

> Do not knock someone else's experience.
>
> —Jace

When Ruth Benedict famously said, "The purpose of anthropology is to make the world safe for human differences," she meant that taking on others' perspectives, even for a moment, goes a long way toward compassion and tolerance. The exceptional breastfeeders I interviewed reflect often on their winding, uphill treks toward breastfeeding. Their desire to make the hard-won lessons meaningful forms a strong basis for solidarity.

NONJUDGMENT DAY IS COMING![7]

It is imperative among exceptional breastfeeders to remain nonjudgmental. Amelia, who co-nurses with her transgender lesbian partner, Sami—an arrangement that attracts some negative scrutiny itself—started to say, "Some people solve [breastfeeding problems] by saying, 'Well, we're just going to formula-feed.' I think that is awful." She immediately corrected herself: "No, I don't think that is awful. People make whatever choices they are going to make." She intended her critique about choosing formula not as a censure of other parents but rather as a commentary on the less than ideal circumstances that make formula the default option. She and her partner both favored an explicitly feminist stance that refused to equate mothering practices with morality (or with gender, for that matter). Instead, like many of the breastfeeders I interviewed, Amelia specified that her breastfeeding decisions were right *for her*. The choices were "right" in Amelia's family because both parents were "able to have that relationship with [their son]," not because their choices were the only good ones.

Amelia was especially loath to cast judgment on anyone else. She said of the "judgy, sneaking aspects" of others' interactions with her and Sami, "It is harder for me not to notice the little cues that people are trying to make at you." The two agreed that Sami was better able to "tune it out" when others leveled microaggressions in their direction. Sami and Amelia, even though they are in the same family, weathered different challenges in coming to their strong sense of solidarity with other parents. Sami said, "I don't always see all of the sideways glances and stuff. I just shut it out. I wonder too if it might be sort of my history. I have the experience of being so incredibly uncomfortable in my body in public. Not for the past decade, but having that in my past of having transitioned, I wonder if that makes me sort of really glad for the experience of not feeling ashamed of that. I wonder if it is just a perspective thing on it. That sort of helps me be more like, 'Fuck it.'" Sami's thick skin deflected negative judgment. Amelia, on the other hand, repeatedly pushed back against judgmental others—including medical providers and some of their extended family members. This exhausting and unwelcome work became something of a consciousness-raising exercise; nobody else, she thought, should have to deal with these barriers just to feed and care for their children. She often chose not to stay silent, which would have been the easier option in just getting through the day, because she wanted to pave a clearer course for those who come after her.

Exceptional breastfeeders like Amelia make the case that bottles and formula are fine options if they are truly and freely chosen options. Low supply, discomfort with breastfeeding, scheduling or sleep problems, suck reflex difficulties, and anatomical differences are among the many presumably "legitimate" reasons not to breastfeed. (Winnie, a lactation support layperson, differentiates "legitimate" reasons from those based on misinformation or lack of hands-on support—for example, never getting help correcting a poor latch.) Valerie tried to understand why some women do not breastfeed, ultimately posing the rhetorical question, "Why does society make it so hard?"

The breastfeeders I talked to know that breastfeeding success hinges on having unfettered access to the necessary support. Reflecting on how she was able to manage where others do not, Valerie hedged:

> This isn't something I would say to anybody except the breastfeeding sociologist, but I am awesome. I deserve a medal. I am so proud of the fact that we have never used a single drop of formula in this house ever. All of my babies have been absolutely, 100 percent exclusively breastfed, nothing but breast milk until they are six months old and continuing on nursing until they are at least twelve months; twenty-four months is my ultimate goal. We did it with one. It was my choice to stop at the other two, I guess. I feel a little bit like I failed with those two, honestly. But I am so proud of myself, and I feel like if, as a working mom, I can do it, other women can do it. And a little like *I understand, after having all of the trouble with my second one* [emphasis added], I understand how you can be at the point where you want to give it up. . . . I get it, on the one hand; but on the other hand, I don't get it. Only because my experience has been overall pretty supported. Besides some physical issues, I've never had any trouble. Even being a working mom, I am so blessed to be at a big company who is usually supportive of breastfeeding mothers, and I've really had an easy time with breastfeeding. It's not just because I'm awesome. [Laughs]

"All the trouble" that Valerie encountered in breastfeeding her second child brought about her awareness that others may have good reasons to stop breastfeeding. Her feelings about her own breastfeeding, which toggled between pride and failure, reflected American individualism. She sounded like a neoliberal conservative, and she was. She took responsibility and credit for her choices and then wondered aloud why other mothers could not manage the same success. But upon consideration of the troublesome time she had breastfeeding one of her children, she seized on the fact that social supports made a substantial difference. It follows that those who do not have the same advantages are unlikely to have such an "easy time with breastfeeding." This realization—that structural barriers (and oppression), perhaps more than individual shortcomings, are to blame for many breastfeeding struggles—is the point of origin for unity and solidarity.

MASSAGING THE MESSAGE

"He's eating from a bottle, and that is an OK way to eat," Marnie corrected a friend for the benefit of the friend's three-year-old. The friends, each with a child in tow, bumped into one another at their farm share pickup location and got to talking. The three-year-old, confused, asked his mother, "Why is he eating from a bottle?" His mother imprudently replied, "Because Marnie's boobies are broken." This was too much. Marnie understood that breastfeeding is now normal to small children in certain circles and that this profound gain is a communal point of pride. But the friend's explanation to the toddler negated the value of Marnie's experience (not to mention the silly and slanderous claim about Marnie's body). Marnie objected to the "idea that everyone should always, at all costs to themselves, have their baby breastfeed." Though breastfeeding became important to Marnie personally, she resented on others' behalf the "distressing and prevailing attitude" that everyone must breastfeed. At a hospital-sponsored infant care class she and her partner enrolled in, she observed, "The whole message was, 'You should breastfeed; if you don't breastfeed you are a bad mother.'" Breastfeeding advocates who mean to be supportive and informative can come off as judgmental and controlling, particularly when they fail to take special circumstances—like adoption, surrogacy, IGT, gender nonconformity, and same-sex parents—into account or make normative assumptions instead of aiming for maximum inclusivity.

Dogmatic positions do not sit well with exceptional breastfeeders, who know that their own unusual takes on mothering tasks might be next to come under fire. For example, Marnie took the time to think about how the infant care training that she observed might impact others in a variety of circumstances: "Maybe formula is not the ideal thing to give your newborn, but it is the practical reality for a lot of women—especially in two-parent households where there are two earners, where there are lower income families, where if you're working at McDonald's, they are not exactly going to give you enough time to pump every time you need to. I think La Leche League comes from a very immense place of privilege in how they talk about formula and how they talk about feeding and nursing and nurturing children."

It takes some awareness to develop this degree of empathy. Exceptional breastfeeders might recognize the parallels of their own struggles to those of other parents. Unlike the lactation leaders and breastfeeders who enjoy the unexamined privilege to be able to vocally reject formula as inferior as they stay home with their babies and nurse on demand, Marnie was hyperaware of "practical realities." Her own intervening circumstances involved the physiological (and scheduling) dilemmas with inducing lactation, volatile breastfeeding disagreements within her intimate partnership, and the external demands of her full-time job. She named her privileges in being able to breastfeed where others might not have all the same options open to them.

Amy took a more liberal philosophy in offering breastfeeding support under the auspices of LLL. She explained, "I feel the group that my colleagues and I run, we are pretty open, welcoming, respecting of a lot of variety of mothering types. But I feel like some groups can be very hard-nosed and straitlaced, but I think that's based more on the leader, not necessarily the organization. So I don't ding the organization for that because I think it has to do with leaders. They mean well, and they really want to help, and they put a lot of effort into it."

Amy, who fed her baby both breast milk and formula, strived to welcome those who were feeding their babies in all different ways. At the same time, she defended the good intentions of both LLL and the "very hard-nosed" leaders. Though giving everyone the benefit of the doubt was important to her (probably a good quality considering that she is a tax fraud investigator!), she did not let them off scot-free. Amy saw problems with their narrow perspective, remembering comments that were "ridiculous" and "stupid," and then made her own efforts to combat the traditional LLL idea that formula is almost never necessary.

The newer rule of thumb "fed is best," fails to fully capture the flipped script that Amy sought to promote, however. Under the guise of preventing horrific (though rare) cases of "infant starvation," this phrase became a gauntlet thrown down at the feet of breastfeeding advocates. The Fed Is Best Foundation, started in 2016 by Christie del Castillo-Hegryi, a mother and medical doctor, replaces the scare tactics attributed to breastfeeding advocates, portrayed as one-dimensional, aggressive proselytizers, with scare tactics of its own. Representatives of the current version of "fed is best" repeatedly suggest on the foundation website and in numerous op-ed pieces—despite only having what the American Council on Science and Health suggests is paltry, speculative evidence[8]—that waiting to feed a newborn until the breastfeeder's milk comes in can lead to a host of spectrum disorders like autism and attention deficit disorder (which research tenuously connects to newborn jaundice). As we see in the antivaccination community,[9] many middle-class parents harbor singular fears about these behavioral disorders and blame bad medical protocols for unfairly superseding what they see as instinctual, naturalistic parenting. The storyline coming from "fed is best" is especially effective because it already exists. The difficulty with this narrative, if it succeeds in convincing easily frightened caregivers, is that breastfeeders will be more and more likely to give up their goals (just as parents delay or forgo vaccination). It is a potential overcorrection to the apocryphal breastfeed-or-bust mentality in which parents are supposedly willing to let their babies starve rather than provide formula when necessary. Continuing to breastfeed *will* bring about enough colostrum in the early days and, eventually, a sufficient milk supply in most cases.

Overbearing lactivists exist of course, as Marnie attested, but the exceptional breastfeeders I talked to carefully avoided the reductive messages of "breast is best" or "fed is best." The message exceptional breastfeeders like Amy want to send is more like, "Do your best," or—if that puts too much of the onus on blame-prone mothers—perhaps, "Do what is best for you and your family under the circumstances." This last sentiment, by the way, is one that exceptional breastfeeders sing in chorus.

Breastfeeders get on board with a shared message by virtue of having contact (online or in person) with parents who experience different challenges. An effect of seeking inspiration is that exceptional breastfeeders' perspectives may shift when they read of others' travails. Sabine, for her part, renewed her dedication to milk donation after witnessing one baby's health improve on donor milk. She said, "To see him now—we've kept in touch—he's a beautiful, perfect little baby. They would bring him to the donors if anybody in the family was sick to nurse directly so that we would make the right antibodies for him." For Sabine, seeing was believing. And this belief in the healing power of breast milk led to action in solidarity and support of other families. These actions both shape and reflect more inclusive attitudes toward a broader variety of infant feeding and care practices.

PLAYING OUT CONTROVERSIES

Before I lead a round of "Kumbaya," it is important to remember the messy social discourse that sometimes allows for consensus and other times only increases divisions. Exceptional breastfeeders are well aware of the competing ideologies and controversial clinical practices surrounding breastfeeding. Often, when they do take on others' perspectives, engage in networking, or seek inspiration in others' stories, they cannot avoid immersion into all of the charged controversies. Online and in-person breastfeeding support groups and the like provide venues for some of these controversies to play out. Exceptional breastfeeders observe and participate in these dramas—what sociologist Erving Goffman calls *dramaturgical action*,[10] acting for others to see and judge positively—and arrive at conclusions. They stake their positions in ways that feel right and that balance their babies' needs, their own identities, and their social contribution.

Ellen is among several exceptional breastfeeders I interviewed who tangled with LLL bureaucracy. Upon discovering that Ellen gave her baby formula as a supplement to breastfeeding, an LLL representative warned her, "Oh, well, I don't know if [the application to become a leader] is going to go through so well anymore." Ellen said, "That made me feel really, really crappy because this whole experience was about me putting a baby to my breast when I wasn't breastfeeding anymore and relactating. This is what made me so passionate. And they were kind of going off, saying because I had formula-fed that I didn't qualify to be a La Leche League leader."

The exceptional quality of her breastfeeding is what made her passionate about breastfeeding advocacy in the first place. The red tape prompted her to go another route, enrolling in a maternal care graduate program. The overly dogmatic LLL policy felt like a personal affront to Ellen, who would have been an avid proponent for the organization. This emotional experience fired her up. She doubled down on her commitment to helping others breastfeed in whatever way they could, if they wished to do so.

Controversies show up relentlessly in the online realm. There are many more people, and some of them ignore the rules of politeness that usually prevail in face-to-face social interactions. Strict moderators and strong user guidelines can create more civil environments, even if it is an uphill battle. BWDBF requires approval for all posts, which ensures that the content aligns with the group's values, but then volunteer moderators have to

monitor the comments. And sometimes a controversial post will be captured and reposted elsewhere, which could leave it open to attack. Allies
might then traffic to those new online locations and defend the original
author or the particular breastfeeding practice (such as extended nursing, breastfeeding in public or in online pics, sleep sharing, milk sharing,
or wet-nursing). These defense maneuvers usually come from individuals,
but sometimes groups launch organized counterstrikes. I observed one
feminist-oriented Facebook group coordinate visits to another breastfeeding advocacy site, where they planned to systematically denounce recent
posts in which authors made TERF (trans-exclusionary radical feminist)
arguments. The online comrades then returned to their home group and
analyzed the reactions, naming individual offenders (which is why my
discussion here is vague on specific details; I do not wish to reveal identities). Anyone reading these threads gets exposure to the various ideological
battles surrounding breastfeeding. They can see all sides, ask questions if
they want, and come to their own conclusions.

Considering others' honest questions broadens perspectives. Months
after our interview, Cricket, a former milk donor, emailed me to ask if I had
any contributions to offer a member of an online moms' group. Apparently
a potential peer milk donor posted to ask if anyone else had shared milk,
explaining that her "mom brain" was keen to do it but that her "lawyer brain"
wondered about liability. This question had never before come to my attention. I suppose I just had never encountered any lawyers, because this concern seems an obvious sticking point. What if one's donated milk caused an
allergic reaction for a stranger's infant? Maybe the donor forgot to disclose
a medication or dairy-rich diet, for instance? I can imagine liability worries
curtailing the practice or encouraging official monitoring. Is informal milk
sharing an irresponsible Wild West where anything goes or a do-it-yourself
Shangri-la of neighborly unity that sticks it to the man? These are the sorts
of questions that caregivers consider among themselves in their internet
discussions.

The contradictory meanings of milk rise to a fever pitch with milk sharing. Here, milk becomes altruistic and life-giving on the one hand, and yet
it seems like risky and potentially lethal on the other.[11] A couple of survey
studies of informal milk sharing in the United States found that the vast
majority of recipients engage in some degree of risk assessment and donor

screening and that knowing the person probably cuts down on concerns that the milk might be contaminated or of poor quality.[12] In my more limited observations, donors also screen recipients, sometimes to be sure their needs are legitimate and also to assess whether they are trustworthy in general. They do this work subtly. Donors may not think of what they do as "screening" when they reach out to their personal networks first or when they scroll through strangers' online requests and select one to contact. Loud public commentary on the "safety" of the milk can seem irrelevant to these players because they know that *they* engaged in these practices on a foundation of trust. Perhaps some other people shared milk blindly, but not them.

There are limits to forging solidarity from social media interactions exclusively. Online worlds can be echo chambers in which our own opinions reverberate back to us, limiting our exposure to differing points of view. This phenomenon certainly happens with some exceptional breastfeeders; those immersed in crunchy worlds share a general distrust of conventional medicine and its motives. These exceptional breastfeeders feel in sync with one another about what is right and expected within the same value system. Ariel offered this fundamental refrain: "It's not that I would judge a mother for giving formula, but just personally my choice is that I would do anything I can to give my daughter breast milk." Her tone was not judging (someone can easily make this sort of statement in which they are very much *are* judging). Still, she also stood by her choice not to give formula, which her circumstances allowed. The controversial aspects of her breastfeeding (doing "anything" to give breast milk) further bonded Ariel with other exceptional breastfeeders.

RECIPROCITY

"I feel like dirt for asking," confessed Rita, a nurse who insisted that milk donors provide their bloodwork before she would accept their milk for the baby she adopted. She explained that she is well aware that her request is on the onerous side: "I'm on Human Milk for Human Babies, and I see all the stuff." "All the stuff" refers to the online conversations and debates about pasteurizing milk to ensure its safety and how mothers trust other mothers without the medical proof. She felt "like dirt," she said, because "you are doing this nice thing for me, but at the same time, reality being what it is, I'd like to see that you are HIV-negative." Her internal conflict highlights one example of the many unwritten rules of reciprocity. In this case, Rita had to set aside rules of politeness in order to keep her parenting conscience clear. She counted on at least some of the other breastfeeders to understand and to be charitable enough to go to the trouble of obtaining medical tests. (Some did.)

Exceptional breastfeeders, especially those who share milk, donate to milk banks, or co-nurse, constantly negotiate and reaffirm reciprocity rules. And they do so in ways that build community. In response to a neighbor's urgent online request for breast milk, several local women offered to pump or to share their freezer stash. One woman chimed in with this quintessential comment: "I just want to say how awesome this thread is!! You all are so lucky to give liquid gold to this baby! My kids are weaned or else I'd pump for you!! I love our village of moms." Everyone wins in this framing. The rules are not set by medical authorities or by any legal protocols, though preexisting social nuances matter. And this sort of cheerleading makes milk sharing and co-nursing seem not only acceptable and gratifying but also important community work.

GIFT-GIVING

"I've *given*; it sounds so weird to say *donated*," insisted Jen about pumping her extra milk for several friends, family members, and acquaintances. She tried unsuccessfully to estimate how much milk she had given over the past few years. She knew that she had filled other families' chest freezers several times and that she pumped daily for specific infants (and nursed them on occasion). She thought of her milk as a gift, and she would not monetize or estimate the value of that heartfelt impulse; that meant she did not count the bags or the ounces or the precise numbers of freezers full. Jen probably disliked *donation* because it suggests too impersonal a gift, like cutting a check or dropping off unwanted household items at Goodwill.

In the early days of milk donation (in the first half of the twentieth century), the donors received payment.[13] Breast milk became both "giftified" and commodified after that point, as society began constructing the sub-stance as sacred and as "good parenting in a bottle," for which the milk banks had to charge.[14] Jen's imprecision placed the milk comfortably in the gift category. She did not keep score because her generosity was genuine. Ignoring the quantity meant that nobody could attach a monetary value. Her work did not go unnoticed. Not only were the recipients grateful, but Jen also became a role model, inspiring others to donate milk too.

Breast milk's high value makes its exchange even more of a delicate social maneuver than it otherwise might be. Many people consider breast milk to be an intimate substance since it is a product of the maternal body. Some of the breastfeeders I interviewed felt squeamish about milk donation for this reason. Marilyn, for instance, referred to media reports on scientific findings that suggest one's body tailors breast milk ingredients and fat con-tent specifically to the individual needs of the gestational mother's baby. This involuntary physiological intelligence, she implied, undermines the whole enterprise of milk sharing. "Mother's milk" exists for the mother to give to *her* baby, some say. Even some donors who do not ascribe to this milk-specificity idea feel that there is some implied intimacy in breast milk sharing—including in the milk itself. So giving it to someone is an intimate practice. Gift-giving and receiving already create a delicate negotiation; this intimacy only magnifies the situation.

I have personal qualms about asking for gifts; I suppose I harbor a fear of asking too much of others. I never could enroll myself in a gift registry or tell my partner what I want for my birthday. Lucky for me and for my babies, my inability to ask for milk donations did not preclude others from giving me their extra. Similarly, when Sabine discerned that a friend was wary about asking for milk, she strongly corrected the friend: "Are you kidding me!" Of course she wants to help, she assured her friend. "That's what friends are for," said Sheena, another mother, who nursed a friend's baby.

Some donors I talked to for this project worried a little about initiating an offer. Rhonda wanted to give milk to a friend but felt unsure about how it would be received—it is not the norm, after all, and she did not want to overstep the bounds of their friendship. The risk was that her friend might think that Rhonda was being weird by offering this intimate gift. She recalled, "Her baby wasn't really gaining weight, and the pediatrician was pushing her to supplement and she hadn't yet. But I asked—I said, 'I have a lot of milk. If you want, you can have it.' I didn't really know if she would take it or not, but she was like, 'Oh, my God, that would be awesome; I'll totally take it.'"

In a display of etiquette, Rhonda downplayed the gift by pointing out that she had "a lot of milk," which could mean in her freezer or just that she regularly produced more than enough. Social rules make it seem rude or overly familiar to give too generous a gift. The reality of milk donation sometimes means extra time spent pumping, a need for more supplies like bags for the milk, delivery or shipping costs, maintenance and cleaning of the pump and its parts, and a depletion of calories that have to be replaced. It is not socially appropriate for donors to complain about these inconveniences. But milk donation gets complicated at times. Milk donors want to know where their valuable milk is going.

THE DESERVING POUR

"We think she might be selling the milk," came the warning in Adriana's inbox. Some other members of the website Human Milk for Human Babies (HM4HB), for which Adriana served as a volunteer moderator, became suspicious when they kept seeing the same request for milk donations:

> "Fran" was on a couple of other pages, like a couple of cloth diapering pages, where she was telling people that she was a deaf lady, Army wife, that was in an abusive relationship. I think she had four or five kids. She had this whole sob story, and it would go on. I think a couple of people had gone on onlythebreast .com, which is a milk-selling website, and she was on there. I don't know for sure if she was selling mine, but she seemed very nice on the text message. I never met her. I left it on my porch, and she came and got it.

Adriana, reluctant to malign milk sharing outright, described the whole scenario as a "semibad experience." She said, "I know that when it happens that it makes you very leery. Because I could have donated it to someone who really needed the milk." Adriana had two concerns: (1) that the gift of milk had been "wasted" by going to someone who obtained it under false pretenses and who was not going to use it in the way in which it was intended (to nourish her own needy baby) and (2) that this isolated incident might turn others away from milk donation. Politicians and WIC employees air familiar-sounding hostile worries that poor women might sell the formula that they obtain for free.[15]

Adriana quickly added that after the dubious donation—she left room for doubt because she was not absolutely certain that the woman was lying—she had a redeeming, positive experience donating forty ounces to a "mom . . . for her baby." She highlighted this contrasting experience because it was something that she could feel good about and because she wanted to garner support for informal milk sharing. Sure, there are occasional one-off bad interactions, but that is no reason to deny milk to the many deserving families out there, she suggested. If potential donors or recipients fixate on the rare negative experience, the entire social project could collapse like a house of cards. Future caregivers would not want to risk participation.

But there is a big difference between clearing out the freezer stash and going to the trouble to pump milk for a particular needy family. Susan explained, "It's not like it was with [my first son] where I just ended up with extra milk in the process of taking care of my baby. But [pumping for a specific family] is something that I'm doing intentionally, and it is taking away from my family and my own time and my own life." Although she added, "I'm glad to be doing it. It's important to me," Susan wanted to underscore this distinction because it drove her choices about to whom she would donate. Kelly demonstrated less concern about her milk's destination. She called the milk bank in her state "because they will take it. They have to have it tested and stuff. I don't remember the results. I just remember it got out of my freezer, and I felt like I didn't throw it away. That was good." Rhonda Shaw, who also studies breastfeeding, considers the symmetry and asymmetry in breast milk sharing and co-nursing relations.[16] The duration, the degree of labor investment, and the quality of the relationship between the caregivers all figure into the relative power dynamics. At one end of the spectrum, donating to the milk bank quickly shuts out the donor mother, and after the clinic sterilizes the milk—literally and figuratively—the milk belongs to the recipient mother.[17] The person who pumped the milk is no longer part of the social relationship. At the opposite pole, each individual's perception and experience of breastfeeding figures prominently.

Eve tried to donate through onlythebreast.com in hopes of helping women who could not afford the milk bank (at $3–5 per ounce), but this grieving mother gave up after fielding numerous requests from fetishists, who boldly asked her to nurse them, and dealing with twenty to twenty-five men who "tried to trick [her]" into giving them her milk by posing as mothers.[18] She responded to the frank requests (versus those committing subterfuge) with a nonjudgmental "That's just not something that I am into." But the milk bank would take it, and the milk bank could be trusted. Kerry and Eve had little interest in tracking their milk from that point. Just a generalized sense of having contributed to many babies and caregivers was sufficient.

Ariel skipped the milk bank option because peer donation seemed more "charitable"; she appreciated that families did not have to go through any hoops to get the milk and that they did not have to pay for it. She liked knowing their stories. Valerie said that she donated to individuals because "it makes me feel good to meet the actual people. And of course they are grateful. . . . I love meeting with babies and looking at their chubby thighs and thinking that I helped with that too." Along this scale of largesse, all the donors wanted the milk they worked for to be put to the best use possible.

But there are differing interpretations about the relative value of giving to milk banks versus informal milk sharing. Millicent noted, at one extreme, that there is "a finite amount of milk at the milk bank" but that "if the mom is having surgery . . . or is just having a long delay in her milk coming in . . . you can make that emotional hard time a little bit easier by donating milk." She said, "If I had excess or if I make excess, then why not give it to some-one else who needs it?" Millicent gave to individuals because they needed it and because milk banks could not fulfill all the need out there. She too characterized her donation as emotional support, an apt reminder that milk is profoundly meaningful.

Susan did both milk bank donations and peer-to-peer milk sharing. She explained, "Informal milk sharing has its own value too, but when it's the milk bank, it's equivalent to organ donation because of the lives it saves." She should know. Susan and her family felt comforted when they donated their deceased daughter's heart valves. The formalized donation also enables medical service providers to carefully monitor the milk's safety, triage its use via the standards by which they dispense it, and provide the life-saving substance to as many babies as possible. The analogy to organ donation effectively normalizes this expert surveillance and secures breastfeeding as a medical matter.[19] Though organ donation is still thought to be a "gift," it is not the kind that nurtures relationships.[20] Milk bank donation cuts out the relationship element with mothers and other caregivers and turns the milk into medicine.

With the more personal informal donations, the potential for social discomfort increases along with the potential for meaningful social connection. Remember Valerie's pride in others' babies with chubby thighs. Not only do many think that donated milk should be needed,[21] but some donors expect recipients to amply demonstrate that need. Susan's utter commitment to pumping and donating was motivated by her beliefs that "every baby deserves breast milk. And every mother deserves being able to feed her baby breast milk." But because supply is limited, she said, "You have to prioritize. So my priority was just for the baby's sake. You know, my gift to these babies. It would . . . be less likely I would donate if the baby wasn't having any health issues, and the older the baby, the less necessary the breast milk would be. Somebody who is just like, 'I just want some extra milk for my twelve-month-old,' isn't going to be as compelling to me as somebody who has a newborn whose mother was drug-addicted, and they're taking care of a foster baby, this drug-addicted baby." Susan could provide generously to a needy baby much more readily than she could a mother looking to supplement already adequate nutrition. Like some other donors I interviewed, she scanned the requests on the breast milk sharing websites, looking for the most compelling story. Successful recipients grasp this unspoken rule and detail their circumstances in private messages and emails that they send to those they know have extra milk. Others post public pleas like this one: "My son is needing a milk donation. He is allergic to formula. He is two months old. When he was one week, I had to go into surgery. . . . As my recovery progresses, I have peaks in my pain and my milk supply reduces dramatically. This is my third request. At one month my son was underweight due to him getting seriously ill for two weeks. Thanks to the milk that has been given to us, he is a healthy, chubby baby boy." It appears important to convince donors of the child's need and to prove that the caregiver has already made every reasonable attempt to breastfeed and/or increase supply. The mother quoted above—and there are thousands of posts just like it—indicated that without the milk, her baby could lose his gains. She cited many unforeseen and unpreventable events like her surgery, the baby's illness, the difficult milk production, and the formula allergy. Another prospective recipient might have less luck inducing donors to help if she asked for milk because returning to work has slowed her supply or because she wants some milk for an older baby. These are not the kinds of reasons that wrench hearts.

This hierarchy of need, repeated in multiple posts across many sites, makes for a pattern that helps construct the rules of exchange. A woman posted this response to someone's offer of frozen milk: "I would love some! I have low supply due to an autoimmune disease, and while we're almost to one year, my heart breaks a little thinking of not being able to give her breast milk. If there are younger babies in need, please give it to them. If there is any left we would be so happy to have it and it would mean we could make it to one year!" She understands that her child's "need" is lower than that of a younger baby. Her statements also reveal that at least part of the reason she wants the milk is to fulfill some emotional and symbolic needs. She wants to reach the arbitrary and proverbial one-year goal, and she needs to mend her broken heart caused by thinking of her own inadequacy. This compelling reason she provides is in hopes of getting leftovers, assuming that this use of the milk is better than throwing it away (or, maybe, having it made into breast milk jewelry—yes, that is a thing).[22]

A few donors told me that they preferred being able to peruse public posts over receiving direct requests that are painful to turn down. It feels discourteous and even selfish to say "no" to someone directly. The donors reading through global requests could set their own criteria (e.g., "need," location, timing, LGBT status) or even choose to respond to the post that hits them the hardest emotionally. Peggy said, "It stuck with me a little bit more," when she read online that a mother with cancer needed breast milk for her infant. Recipients with less dramatic stories to offer may struggle to find donors.[23]

Milk sharing within one's existing social network can be less fraught. Jessica donated milk to friends of friends when she experienced oversupply with her first nursling. She had trouble with supply with her second child, so she returned to that network, feeling confident about directly asking individuals if they had extra milk. They knew her history of donating to others in their circle and would almost certainly view Jessica as deserving. And when Dorinne, who worked in maternity, announced her coming adoption, friends and coworkers immediately said, "I have milk! I have milk!" They started dropping off coolers full of frozen bags at her house long before the baby arrived. Like a meal train in celebration of the arrival of a new community member, milk sharing can be a giving ritual, a part of a system of generalized reciprocity, in which all community members are potential participants and beneficiaries. Everyone pitches in when they can without thought of immediate or direct repayment.

Donors rarely demand displays of gratitude. Kerry passed along milk along with hand-me-downs. She reasoned with the milk recipient, "You don't have enough [milk], and I have too much, so let me help me you." Mira received such a generous donation that she could not believe it:

> So I met her in the Old Navy parking lot, and I get there and we exchange coolers, and I get home, and as I am starting to go through the ounces and I am calculating stuff. There was close to 800 ounces. So I called her up: "Did you realize you gave me way more? Did you need this back?" Because I knew she was working. She was like, "No, no, no, no, I realized it was more. I just wanted to get it cleaned out. It is fine." And so I called my husband at the time just in tears, and he was like, "What? Is everything OK with the baby?" And I said, "No, it is great!" I think he thought I had totally gone off my rocker. [Laughs]

Mira's tearful gratitude contrasted with the donor's air of nonchalance. It was really not a big deal to clear out her freezer and then drive a few miles to meet at a convenient drop-off, the donor insisted to Mira. Another of Mira's donors "ended up with a huge oversupply. She had her freezer full in her garage, her freezer full [in her house], her mother-in-law's freezer full, and her mother's freezer full." Mira was doing *her* a favor.

A study of French milk donors found that most (60 percent) donated because they had extra milk and the rest (40 percent) were motivated by an interest in helping out other mothers.[24] The two reasons probably overlap. Adriana minimized her donations, saying it was a win-win proposition in which her freezer got emptied, she got relief from engorgement, and she got to help someone else. Yesenia, among other donors I talked to, did not remember all of her donations. These donors who use the online milk-sharing networks Eats on Feets and HM4HB may not keep score or encourage much ritual. When the relationship is momentary, casual, and uneventful, donors (and, to a lesser degree, grateful recipients) tend to forget the specifics. But they participate in a bigger social project. Yesenia really cared about milk donation as a concept even if she spent little time thinking about who exactly received her milk. These broad connections can be even more poignant and political when milk sharing and other kinds of exceptional breastfeeding help build queer families, support black women in reclaiming their mothering legacy, or welcome an adoptive or foster baby into the breastfeeding community.

MISSED CONNECTIONS, MEANINGFUL CONNECTIONS

Even though donors do not require much in the way of thanks, they are understandably bothered by "flakiness" on the part of uncommunicative recipients, and they can be offended when their milk offers get declined. Rhonda lamented being on the "sorry, we don't want your milk" list at her regional milk bank. She tried donating her milk to a researcher in Boston who never bothered to call her back. (She considered not participating in the present study because of the prior bad experience with researchers.) Her frustrated attempts to donate her milk annoyed her enough to endure the "pain of the drain"—throwing out her milk to make room for food in her small New York City apartment refrigerator. Valerie and Yesenia both mentioned that the onerous criteria of their area milk banks contributed to their choice to go with informal milk donation. The foster care rules against co-nursing irked Margaret, and she felt hurt by their unwillingness to place a baby with her once she obtained legal clearance to be a wet nurse in her state. "There were no takers [of my milk]," she said with regret. The "weird criteria" of the local LLL chapter frustrated Olivia, who thought that they adhered too narrowly to their doctrines.

Of course, I only interviewed those who persisted through these missed connections, but their experiences point to a consistent theme. Rather than only being valuable as a commodity, donated breast milk's real value comes from its intimacy. It is an offering from a loving and dedicated parent to another and/or to another's baby. Many of the donors talked about how poorly they would have felt as a mother if they could not get breast milk for their baby. Thus it is not merely a question of medical or nutritional need. One's identity and fitness as a mother, as a good parent, are in question. Adriana commended another mother for all the pumping she did and all the time she must surely spend looking for donors to supplement her mea-ger supply. She offered the milk in solidarity with these efforts. Likewise,

Jeri and Allie felt for a mother who was struggling to keep up with breast-feeding twins, and the couple went to some trouble to get her some milk. Stories abound about the many recipients who could not breastfeed due to cancer or other severe illness or injury. Sabine talked about one of her milk recipients who had to take medicine to "stay healthy and alive." The medicine passes into breast milk, which prevented the woman from nursing her baby. These blameless others need help from the community's good Samaritans.

Some donors focused more on helping babies rather than other parents, viewing their milk as the vital ingredient that would transform a deprived baby into a thriving one. Hazel, for instance, enjoyed her wet-nursing role as a "community chest." And plenty of donors thought of the milk as valuable in both ways. Ellen donated to the preemies at the neonatal intensive care unit (NICU) who "really need [the milk]." But her concern was not just for the infants. The milk bank forwarded thank-you letters from the grateful mothers, which moved Ellen emotionally. Not incidentally, she decided to become an IBCLC (International Board Certified Lactation Consultant) herself to help others breastfeed. The commitment can be a permanent one. And the intent is often tender and heartfelt, even with casual donations. As a result, having one's milk rejected can feel like a little bit like unrequited love.

To be sure, in certain contexts, reciprocation and even remuneration can be appropriate. Rosemary's acquaintance started a milk-sharing collective in her hippie-ish homeschooling, cloth diapering, slow food movement–loving community. When her oversupply got out of hand with the third child, Rosemary called to say, "I have so much extra milk, and I would love to share it." The friend connected her to a mother who could not breastfeed due to a medication. The recipient reciprocated in small, meaningful—but ultimately unnecessary—ways: "It was really sweet because she would bring me food, muffins, or cabbage, or just something that she had." Rosemary did not require these gifts, but she appreciated that giving them helped the *recipient* feel good about getting the milk: "She always felt like I was giving her milk, that she should give me something. She would give me some food from her farm box . . . and at the end of our journey, I don't know how much milk I gave her, but I donated for many months, maybe three or four months; she gave me a gift certificate to Rainbow Grocery, which is a natural grocery food place because she wanted to show me that she cared for all the milk that I gave her baby." In one sense, Rosemary saw herself as having given to the baby, and babies are not expected to show their thanks. She was also giving as a form of community work. Other donors remembered the odd bunch of flowers or tray of baked goods given to them by the caregivers receiving their milk, but these gestures were not expected or even routine.

Although milk obtained via peer networks is rarely bought and sold,[25] there are exceptions. Small gifts and generalized barter arrangements (favors, really) are about all. Tara explained that milk banks are great for "NICU babies, the preemies, and babies who are ill," because the milk may save their lives and because insurance covers the cost. But her baby needed milk too: "Milk bank milk is like five [dollars] an ounce. Who can do that? At, like, thirty ounces a day? Even if you are supplementing with your own milk. Informal is the way to go. We did some childcare for our primary donor. And we just recently just sent her a thank-you gift like a gift card to a local store. But nowhere near what it would cost for us to actually pay for us to get milk bank milk. . . . An individual family that just needs some breast milk, you have to find another way." Like Tara, many caregivers I interviewed understood the role of the milk bank for dire circumstances, and they reasoned that the high cost has to do with the need for testing, pasteurizing, and monitoring of the milk. But others had the idea that milk banks are for-profit ventures. Media reports about a couple of controversial schemes may fuel this misconception. Ambrosia, a private company, paid low-income Cambodian women for their milk and then resold it in the United States.[26] And Medolac, accused of preying on impoverished black mothers in Detroit, purchased their breast milk for the manufacture of a milk product meant for resale to hospitals. Exploitation is the obvious concern; critics worry that these breastfeeders will be unfairly induced to give up the milk that their own babies need. Some of those parents who sell their milk, however, argue that they have an oversupply: Why should they not be paid for their pumping labor?[27] They reject the patronizing interference of activists who suggest that it is socially reprehensible to sell milk.

Some people misunderstand how the official milk banks (members of HMBANA) operate. Several people told me that the milk banks exploit donors by turning around and selling the milk that the banks obtained for free. Milk bank milk is beyond the means of most families and is available only by prescription. Even with a prescription, stock may run low, and a priority system is in place to help the sickest and youngest babies first.

I was able to get the milk for my children with prescriptions from compliant doctors and all of my savings. Emotions guided my decision to give my sons breast milk. Just like any other exceptional breastfeeder, I thought I should try to give my children any kind of head start that I could, even if the science backing breast milk was unclear and the cost was astronomical. My sons would have fared just fine on formula. I could not possibly judge anyone else's decision on this front, as my own choice was an agnostic one; I did not know whether getting the milk was worthwhile or not. Informal milk sharing seems to be a more viable formula-free option. But could free and easy informal milk sharing be a privilege of those caregivers with connections and status? This is the stuff of controversy.

Donors and recipients decide with whom to share based on whatever criteria they choose and within the networks that feel comfortable. Recall the hard line that Ariel took out of necessity, as she made clear: "Even though I have experience as a mother with low supply, I really wanted [my donation] to be medically for the baby's benefit and not for the mother's peace of mind." She was not on a power trip any more than someone who carefully chooses a charity to which to donate their hard-earned money. But giving away her milk was political, purposeful, and contained within a community of caregivers who she deemed deserving.

Recipients also reproduce homogenous social circles. Katie checked out her potential donors on Facebook: "What do they like? What groups are they in? Where did they attend school? . . . Both of them were elementary teachers; I would imagine they had drug testing and background checks. But they were also very outspoken Christians, and they loved the local Christian radio station. They had tons of pictures of their babies being nursed on Facebook. . . . They seem to be really good people."

They were "really good people" mainly because of their apparent values, which aligned with hers; thus, she felt safe accepting their milk. Although none of the caregivers I interviewed expressed any concern about being shut out of milk sharing for their social status, I have observed the occasional online comment to that effect. Queer parents and people of color may worry about having a harder time accessing milk or giving away milk in these informal settings. There are no regulations in place to protect against discrimination. The system operates exclusively on goodwill.

It seems to be working so far. The cross status milk-sharing pattern I observed was remarkably ubiquitous. It was a pleasant surprise to see self-described religious conservatives freely and proudly sharing their milk with queer parents. Their common goals and identities as parents overcome the usual social, political, and religious differences.

For their part, members of marginalized groups do not always try to infiltrate a mainstream that may or may not accept them as valid and fit parents. They may instead close ranks against a hostile political milieu. Whereas milk selling is anathema to many breastfeeding advocates and many rank-and-file milk-sharing breastfeeders,[28] this may be a privileged view. As Ameena Ali, one of the founders of Chocolät Milk explained, poor women help each other out, and these arrangements necessarily involve cash sometimes. Sharing milk is not unlike home-based day cares, in that a parent can provide a service to make ends meet while simultaneously caring for her own children. Someone with an otherwise bothersome oversupply can sell her milk at a fair bargain or barter with a breastfeeder who cannot produce enough. Another win-win.

But this sort of arrangement interferes with middle-class assumptions. In the mainstream culture, something sold is a commodity. The milk becomes a product subject to government inspection, liability, and laws of the marketplace. Such an arrangement taps into hygiene-obsessed middle-class fears of contamination related to poor handling and the risk of profit-motivated adulteration. Onlythebreast.com, the main platform for milk selling now that craigslist.com forbids these transactions, has a bad reputation in the milk-sharing world. Not only does it allow (and profit from) economically disadvantaged lactating parents to sell to milk-desperate families, but it makes space for truly off-kilter uses of breast milk, such as nutritional supplementation for athletes and body builders and sexual fetishes. These last two reasons for ingesting breast milk actively "queer" the substance by questioning and rearranging its meaning as a substance that is both maternal and precious. Breast milk can be a superfood, enhancing the performance of extreme male bodies. It can be a taboo turn-on—again, primarily for men. Australian author Fiona Giles argues convincingly for a liberal ideological and experiential shift when it comes to breast milk.[29] If we could view it as life-giving, as mother-love (and I would add other care-givers here), as sometimes welcome and sometimes intrusive in its abundance, *and* as a normal part of life (to put it plainly), then the many value questions and debates might lose much of their power to cause turmoil.

But breast milk as infant nourishment will continue to have an exchange value if it is in short supply for some. Medolac sells what it disingenuously markets as "co-op donor milk," which is actually a "commercially-sterile"[30] processed human milk product from lactating individuals who *sold* their milk. Banking on the informal milk-sharing belief system, Medolac sells it to hospitals and, according to their website as of May 2017, to individuals who can take it home for their babies. Milk bank representatives worry about both milk selling and informal milk sharing undercutting donations to them. They discourage gray-market transactions with reminders about the enormous unmet need for breast milk in neonatal units.

The milk banks portray themselves as serving the very neediest babies. This niche purpose, however, may be backfiring because it can only serve a small percentage of those who want and need breast milk. The meaningful interpersonal ways of distributing milk—and the informal sharing and, less frequently, wet-nursing—continue. The clinical and scientific approval given to milk banks and their campaigns that pitch mothers helping mothers helps normalize the larger "breast is best" project that underpins exceptional breastfeeding in all its forms. Routinization, medical surveillance, and legal approval demarcate the seemingly risk-free banks, which serve the few, from the more freewheeling, informal, DIY sharing networks, which serve the many.

INTIMATE CITIZENSHIP

> It feels good to do a good thing.   —Valerie, milk donor

> Conversations that look "at the breast" . . . are not private.
> —Linda Blum, *At the Breast: Ideologies of Breastfeeding and Motherhood in the Contemporary United States* (1999)

All breastfeeding is up for debate. The blur between "private decisions" and "public dialogues," where even the most intimate parts of life are everybody's business, led sociologist Ken Plummer to coin the term *intimate citizenship*.[31] Intimate citizenship is another intersection of our social identity along with gender, sexual identity, race, dis/ability, class, and religion. By definition, exceptional breastfeeders occupy a marginal status as citizen-parents. They are breaching norms in one way or another. But within the overlapping circles in the Venn diagram of intensive mothering (or crunchy moms) and community-mindedness, they are as upstanding as they come. Extending this notion of intimate citizenship, I consider how exceptional breastfeeding, including milk sharing, brings caregivers together in solidarity as they make each choice and both feel good about doing it and experience it as the right thing to do.

Latisha bravely defended breastfeeding to her dubious family members. Her aunts and uncles admonished her not to "whip out her breasts" in front of anyone, and her mother, while ostensibly supportive, sometimes pressed her lips together as she looked sideways at Latisha's breastfeeding practices. Latisha even went so far as to donate her milk, a practice that was far outside of their comfort zone. She said, "I believe in the Bible. I believe in God. I believe God created us, and what he created us for was to do work for the greater good, and that is why I feel like this is my way to pay it forward. This is why [I] donate. I mean, I could give money. You can give thanks. But those things are, I don't know, kind of selfish. To give of yourself is totally—and I'm talking about breastfeeding—you have to be available, I mean, on demand. It is the most selfless act you can do, to breastfeed." Latisha positioned her breastfeeding and her breast milk sharing as a religious mandate and as embodied selflessness and generosity. She performed good lactating citizenship outside of formal surveillance, privately offering something more than money. It is part of her essence and part of her spiritual value to give in this way. She further insisted that she was "not perfect," but that she was doing right.

For Gwendolyn, giving her milk away meant an opportunity to perform good citizenship in a way that had always been unavailable to her: "I really appreciated being involved with that, being able to give this resource that I had. I haven't ever had a lot of money. When you can't just write a check for $200 to the Cancer Society or the Sierra Club, but I can give this. I could give this milk to someone. It was really nice for me to feel like finally I have a skill, I am a resource; it is in high demand, and it will be of great benefit to other people." Breastfeeders in general seem to be doing moral work that includes altruism and maternal sacrifice already;[32] milk donation can extend this altruism even further.

Several donors I talked to characterized their donations to strangers and to milk banks as better than giving money to a good cause. Adriana said, "I cannot give tons of money to everybody in the world, but I can do this." In this context, being an overproducer, with the attendant physically painful body betrayal, is recast as body redemption. Like some pregnancy surrogates, they understand their bodies as being put to use for others' well-being.[33] Donors like Gwendolyn and Adriana possessed something unique and highly valuable that they gave away for free as a community service. They could not even know how much good they were doing, but they trusted their efforts to radiate out into the world.

But where they donate makes a difference to what the donors get out of it. Milk banks are more on the clinical and impersonal side. And finding recipients through large sites like HM4HB and Eats on Feets takes away some of the familiarity that people might see with friends or acquaintances sharing milk. It does not rise to the level of anything like the communal mothering that can happen when breastfeeders in the same social circle share milk or nurse one another's children.

Where most donors and recipients do not keep track of the quantity of shared milk—it takes time and it may be seen to lack social grace—some do, for reasons of self-esteem, gratitude, or incentive. Mira, for instance, counted the ounces she received to be sure she had the right amount and did not have to "go out looking for milk." She also kept track in order to document the success of this community effort to benefit her child. Like keeping a list of first gifts in a baby book, it was proof for posterity that so many people cared.

Adriana recounted the stories of each of the many families to whom she donated for a similar reason: to revel in the solidarity. She said, "It was just so amazing to me that I could nourish this other baby. It is so important. There are no chemicals in it like there is in formula. There is nothing better to give your baby than breast milk and . . . to know that I am helping them grow is just phenomenal." The many superlatives—"amazing," "nothing better," "phenomenal"—reveal just how significant milk sharing can be to a donor. A true believer, Adriana was proud of herself, impressed with the qualities of breast milk, and more to the point, thoroughly convinced that milk sharing is a community responsibility.

And it can be convenient. Talking about pumping for donation, Harriet noted, "It was something that I could do so easily in the comfort of my own home. I could do it in my pajamas. . . . Before I even have my breakfast, I have technically saved a life." She wondered at the fact that something she could do so easily could "make a tremendous difference to other people." The payoff for her small trouble was self-respect and a feeling of interconnectedness. She also represented the leading edge: "When I was growing up, the saying in Ireland in the eighties was 'only two types of people breastfeed, Tinkers and teachers.' The poorest of the poor and the moderately educated. Nobody else did it. That is not the thing to do." Her duty was an instrumental one and also normalized breastfeeding values through her visible praxis. Everyone in her Irish village who needed help nursing their babies came to her. Plus the milk bank knew her well. Harriet actively nurtured this vision of herself as an upstanding citizen in her community.

NormalizeBreastfeeding.org markets this impulse in an ad campaign that includes three successive images of a stylized silhouette: a figure nursing, a figure with breast pump bottles at the chest, and a figure nursing with an SNS. The captions read, respectively, "Nurse," "Pump," "Donate," in a simple-to-remember good citizenship directive reminiscent of "Reduce, Reuse, Recycle."

FROM LETDOWN TO UPLIFT

Exceptional breastfeeding could be the beginning of a social movement that crosses borders and bridges divides. Jeff gave credit where it was due: "I think it's so special that he has received a gift—the blessings from like ten to twenty different women, and a piece of them has helped shape who he is." The metaphysical element aside, these milk donors legitimized Jeff's child by participating in his growth. They also welcomed Jeff and his husband into the fold as fellow worthy parents. And we have seen that donors enjoy being charitable and intend their milk to help make kin and to effect social liberation.

Sheena wound up in an even more intimate situation after experiencing chronic low supply: "You feel like you somehow failed in some way. Like my body is not doing what it is supposed to be doing. I also felt that way about childbirth because I ended up with a C-section, so I think there's so much connected to it. I teach women's studies, so it wasn't like my womanhood was associated with it, but . . . it is such a letdown."

As clear as she was about distinguishing between her self-worth as a woman and feelings about being let down by her own body, Sheena still felt lost. But she was soon overcome with relief. It was not any medical service or formula company or milk bank coming to her rescue. It was another mother who reached out with supplemental milk, providing enough when combined with Sheena's and Romy's (Sheena's partner who induced lactation to help) milk. The three of them together, with the help of pumps and freezers and domperidone and an SNS, got the baby fed. Sheena and Romy at their home took turns nursing with baby at the breast and an SNS filled with the friend's milk, and the friend pumped in the privacy of her own home while her baby slept.

Humanity demands reciprocity. When we get a gift, we give one in return, even if that means we "pay it forward" in a generalized way. For exceptional breastfeeders, sometimes that means becoming more active politically, sharing their milk or their breast, providing emotional support in person or online, seeking a maternity-related vocation, or simply striving to understand others. Imani, late in her pregnancy, thought, "Why not give [breastfeeding] a try?" It turned out better than she could have imagined, and she proselytized to her close her friend:

"Are you going to nurse? What are you thinking?" Imani asked.

Her friend replied, "No, it's not for me."

Imani understood and said, "I used to think that, and I was really pleasantly surprised that it wasn't what I thought it was going to be."

"I don't see myself whipping out my boobs and having a baby on it, no," said the friend.

"Give it a try," insisted Imani.

The friend, noncommittal and unenthusiastic, said, "I don't know. I guess I'll talk to my doctor."

To me, Imani concluded, "Nursing isn't for everybody. Some women are just, 'No, I don't like this. This is not for me.'" She accepted this "no" and did not demand a reason. This stance prevails in my conversations with exceptional breastfeeders. They want breastfeeding—in some fashion or another—available to everyone barrier-free but also without undue pressure. They have tired of the stigma associated with every option, and rather than saying everyone *should* breastfeed, they collectively work toward a world where anyone *can* breastfeed.

BREASTFEEDING JUSTICE

Lisette, who breastfed her adoptive daughter, said, "She was sweet. With nursing, she was just inward toward me and the family. I'm glad I got to do that. . . . I know you can bond with a baby with a bottle. *I know you can.* There was just something sweet about [breastfeeding]." This account celebrates the sweetness, the bonding, and the family-building potential of breastfeeding without tearing down bottle-feeders or assuming an essentialist view.

Ethnographer Tanya Cassidy asserts, "Breastfeeding or lactation activism is a quintessentially local movement enjoying global features, with 'lactivists' networking across the world."[34] The experiences of exceptional breastfeeders validate this observation. Their networking differs a little from that of home birth activists because they may well share even more than expertise and perspectives and political connections. Sometimes they share milk.

Self-identified exceptional breastfeeders more generally—to include those engaged in long-term breastfeeding, co-nursing, inducing lactation, tandem nursing, "queer" breastfeeding and milk sharing—persist through a host of extraordinary challenges. As part of this persistence, they contend with oppressive social discourses and the authorities that enforce them. Exceptional breastfeeders who do what they want (or whatever they can manage), instead of what they are told to do, consistently subvert the system. Their embodied refusal to allow their breastfeeding to reflexively confirm gender norms and prescribed roles destabilizes long-held assumptions. If anyone can breastfeed and if breastfeeding can mean many things, it becomes more difficult to circumscribe motherhood and to keep it hierarchical. Exceptional breastfeeders keep expanding their relationships and the meaning of kinship, which dismantles some of the boundaries around the Western family. Some of them disregard the nuclear family ideal built on a mother and baby foundation, innovating and intensifying other kinds of intimate relations.

Breastfeeding is a memorable time in one's life because it can be integral to relationship-building, identity-making, and perspective-changing.
Its importance to those who engage in it makes it a prime site for effect-
ing social change. Exceptional breastfeeders in particular are likely to attach
political significance—of the liberating kind—to the experience precisely
because others question their practices. They reach out for help, and they
reach out to give it.

Breastfeeding justice requires support for all infant-feeding choices, even
as its proponents work to remove the obstacles to breastfeeding. Addressing
breastfeeding disparities cannot only be about identifying "lack of knowledge" among new parents and providing appropriate educational support,
as if caregivers' ignorance explains uneven rates of breastfeeding; retrain-
ing medical service providers, employers, and the court system on how to
be less discriminatory, more culturally competent, and more accommodat-
ing is also necessary yet still not enough. The commercial sphere, journal-
ism and entertainment, and public health campaigns need to consistently
rebrand breastfeeding in ways that steer clear of shaming, but such an effort
would only be a start. Public health work that measures aggregate outcomes
of probreastfeeding initiatives need to include more attention to satisfaction
(and to off-category definitions of breastfeeding)—not only to increase
initiation and duration rates but to recognize that some caregivers' decisions do not need to be "fixed." There are serious concerns about how much
enacting legislation and regulations to encourage breastfeeding would support (or harm) the aims of justice. Risk narratives that might guide the rule
making tend toward mother-blaming; codifying risk could put those who
cannot breastfeed into legally precarious territory. But enforceable rules
that prevent interference in breastfeeding and that maximize caregivers'
autonomy are sorely needed if society wants to truly support breastfeeding.

Exceptional breastfeeders offer an array of fresh perspectives that can be
contradictory. Even a single individual may hold multiple, discordant views
on breastfeeding because they harbor ambivalence or because they have
wide-ranging experiences with breastfeeding—each child brings a different set of challenges and triumphs. As advocates of breastfeeding justice,
we do not have to reduce their complex realities to a narrow set of positions.
To be effective, advocates cannot rely on reasoning that vilifies formula-
or bottle-feeders, essentializes women as mothers, or ranks parents
from good to bad. Instead of taking a hard-line breast is best attitude, or

overreacting to "lactivism," I recommend a hard-line toward multiplying what is possible and toward always supporting more expansive, creative approaches to breastfeeding.

The exceptional breastfeeders I interviewed offer their insights from a place of resistance and with a bent toward solidarity to make the hard work of mothering better and more satisfying for all.

APPENDIX

List of Participants

Name	Age	Sexual identity	Gender identity	Partner status	Occupation	Political affiliation	Religion	Race/ethnicity
Aaliyah	37	heterosexual	woman	married	midwife	liberal	Muslim	black
Adriana	34	heterosexual	woman	married	tax technician	moderate	Catholic	Latina
Alice	42	heterosexual	woman	remarried	teacher	conservative	Baptist	black
Allie	33	bisexual		married	administrative assistant	liberal	ex evangelical	white
Ameena Ali			woman		midwife/educator	n/a	n/a	black
Amelia	32	lesbian	woman	married	hospitality	progressive	none	white
Amy	30	heterosexual	woman	married	accountant	moderate	Baptist	white
Anais	48	heterosexual	woman	married	teacher	progressive	none	white
Ariel	33	heterosexual	woman	married	homemaker	conservative	Catholic	white
Aster	34	heterosexual	woman	married	singer	progressive	Rastafarian /Ethiopian Orthodox	Latina
Aurora	25	lesbian	woman	married	nanny	progressive	ex evangelical	white
Bailey	30	heterosexual	woman	married	firefighter	conservative	Catholic	white
Beth Ann	25	lesbian	woman	married	student	progressive	exevangelical	white
Candace	40	heterosexual	woman	divorced	school counselor	progressive	none	white
Carena	40	heterosexual	woman	single	teacher	conservative	Baptist	black
Connie	35	bisexual	woman	partnered	marketing	liberal	none	white
Cricket	41	heterosexual	woman	married	business	progressive	none	white
Devin	40	lesbian	butch	married	professor	progressive	ex-Mormon	white
Donna	31	heterosexual	woman	married	city planner	libertarian	none	white
Dorinne	43	heterosexual	woman	married	nurse	none	Christian	white
Ellen	25	heterosexual	woman	married	bookkeeper	unknown	unknown	white

Name	Age	Sexuality	Gender	Marital status	Occupation	Political	Religion	Race
Emie	50	heterosexual	woman	unknown	birth educator	unknown	unknown	Latina
Eve	20	heterosexual	woman	married	student	unknown	unknown	white
Francine	38	heterosexual	woman	married	homemaker	conservative	evangelical	white
Gwendolyn	40	heterosexual	woman	married	doula	lefty	Buddhist	white
Harriet	40	heterosexual	woman	single	writer	unknown	unknown	white
Imani	31	heterosexual	woman	separated	doula/ student	liberal	spiritual	black
Jace	36	pansexual	trans	triad	student	moderate	unknown	white
Jeff	50	gay	man	married	business	progressive	exevangelical	white
Jen	31	heterosexual	woman	married	teacher	progressive	Jewish	white
Jeri	42	lesbian	woman	married	account executive	liberal	ex-Lutheran	white
Jessica	40	heterosexual	woman	married	nurse	Democrat	Jewish	white
Joanie	43	lesbian	butch	divorced	programmer	lefty	spiritual	white
Kadijah	38	heterosexual	woman	divorced	homemaker	liberal	agnostic	black
Katie	34	heterosexual	woman	married	homemaker	Tea Party / right of Republican	evangelical	white
Kelly	36	lesbian	middle of spectrum	partnered	occupational therapist	unknown	unknown	white
Kendra	39	heterosexual	woman	divorced	professor	progressive	none	white
Kerry	23	heterosexual	woman	married	homemaker	unknown	unknown	white
Kiki	38	heterosexual	woman	married	life coach	conservative	ex-Mormon	Polynesian
Kris	32	lesbian	butch	married	doula	progressive	none	white
Kylie	31	heterosexual	woman	married	NICU nurse	none	ex-Catholic / "nature and energy"	white
Lanie	50	heterosexual	woman	married	homemaker	moderate	spiritual	white

(continued)

Name	Age	Sexual identity	Gender identity	Partner status	Occupation	Political affiliation	Religion	Race/ethnicity
Latisha	29	heterosexual	woman	divorced	medical technician	unknown	Catholic	black
Lily	28	heterosexual	woman	single	social worker	Democrat	Catholic	Latina
Lisette	60	heterosexual	woman	single	administrative assistant	progressive	Christian	white
Liza	50	heterosexual	woman	divorced	medical technician	unknown	Catholic	white
Lonny	35	heterosexual	woman	married	midwife	liberal	none	white
Mara	42	lesbian	genderqueer	married	alternative health	progressive	none	white
Margaret	54	heterosexual	woman	widowed	lactation counselor	conservative	Catholic	white
Marilyn	42	heterosexual	woman	married	paralegal	moderate	Catholic	black
Marnie	36	queer	high femme	partnered	professor	progressive	Jewish	white
Marybeth	32	lesbian	woman	partnered	hairdresser	unknown	unknown	black
Melanie	33	heterosexual	woman	married	programmer	Democrat	atheist	white
Millicent	37	heterosexual	woman	divorced	entrepreneur	liberal	Catholic	white
Mira	31	heterosexual	woman	divorced	teacher	unknown	ex-Mormon	white
Mona	33	lesbian	woman	partnered	unknown	none	ex-Catholic	Latina
Naheema	39	heterosexual	woman	married	filmmaker	Democrat	African Traditional	black
Olivia	41	heterosexual	woman	partnered	midwife	moderate	none	white
Peggy	34	heterosexual	woman	married	administrative assistant	liberal	none	white
Rachel	31	lesbian	woman	married	professor	progressive	none	white
Rexi	31	queer	fluid, trans	single	teacher	progressive	Jewish	white
Rhonda	36	bisexual	woman	single	nurse	progressive	Jewish	white

Name	Age	Sexual orientation	Gender	Relationship	Occupation	Politics	Religion	Race
Rita	36	heterosexual	woman	married	midwife	conservative	evangelical	white
Rosemary	38	heterosexual	woman	married	nurse	liberal	none	white
Roxanne	35	heterosexual	woman	married	professor	independent	Mormon	white
Sabine	31	heterosexual	woman	married	teacher	unknown	unknown	white
Sami	36	lesbian	butch, fluid	married	nonprofit manager	progressive	exevangelical	white
Sandra	40	lesbian	femme	married	homemaker	progressive	none	white
Shawn	30	bisexual	boyish	partnered	job seeker	progressive	unknown	black / Latina / Asian / Native American
Sheena	36	lesbian	woman	partnered	professor	progressive	Jewish	White
Sheila	51	heterosexual	woman	married	medical assistant / doula	liberal	none	white
Sherry	39	heterosexual	woman	married	nonprofit manager	liberal	unknown	white
Spring	40	heterosexual	woman	married	IT professional	Republican	unknown	white
Stella	41	heterosexual	woman	married	accountant	progressive	unknown	white
Susan	39	heterosexual	woman	married	retail clerk	Republican	unknown	white
Tayshia	42	heterosexual	woman	married	teacher	progressive	none	black
Thad	51	queer	trans	married	medical technician	progressive	unknown	white
Thomas	42	gay	man	married	teacher	moderate	Baptist	white
Tiana	30	heterosexual	woman	married	student	progressive	African Traditional	black
Valerie	38	heterosexual	woman	married	engineer	independent	evangelical	white
Vanessa	44	heterosexual	woman	married	professor	liberal	none	white
Winnie	75	heterosexual	woman	married	administrative assistant	progressive	unknown	white
Yesenia	32	heterosexual	woman	married	law enforcement	Republican	Catholic	Latina

ACKNOWLEDGMENTS

Thank you to all of the generous mothers and others who offered the insights and stories that form the basis for this book.

I also owe a debt to the anonymous reviewer, to Barbara Katz Rothman, and to readers Wendy Simonds, Julia Sinn, Anthony Garcia, Beatriz Reyes-Foster, Susan Falls, Liza Warehouse, Jason Warehouse, Rebecca Nowlin Green, Elroi Windsor, Andrea Riordan, Emilio Mesa, Liz Soluri, and Cherie Barkey. Their suggestions greatly improved this work. Any mistakes or faults in reasoning are entirely my own.

I am grateful to two students, Aurora Barber and Morgan Botelle, for their assistance with transcribing. Thanks to Kendall Silveira for forwarding the original call for participants. The Cabrillo College Federation of Teachers made it possible for me to take a sabbatical from teaching in order to write this book.

I especially wish to thank to my two young children, Evan and Leo, who first inspired me to explore the topic of exceptional breastfeeding. Over the past four years, they waited for my motherly attention while I worked, ironically enough, to finish an interview, analyze a transcript, or conclude a writing session—about motherhood.

NOTES

CHAPTER 1   NURSING IS PUBLIC

1. This term plays on the "ethnographic exception," a basic concept in anthropology that discards the notion that a human behavior is "natural" if it is not a universal practice. For example, Margaret Mead (1935) famously cast doubt on twentieth-century Western beliefs about gender roles by describing cultures in which women were the providers and men were preoccupied with their appearance.

2. Rothman 2007:80.

3. Sociologist Katherine Carroll (2015) calls milk donation "care work" for this reason.

4. Quandt 1995.

5. Blum 1999; Campo 2010.

6. The final episode of the popular HBO series *Girls*, which aired April 16, 2016, dramatizes these prevailing narratives. The main character, Hannah Horvath, worries aloud about her child's future if she pumps her milk instead of "bonding" at the breast. And her best friend, Marnie, openly expresses her disdain for "formula feeders."

7. As author Ayelet Waldman emphasizes in her 2009 memoir *Bad Mother: A Chronicle of Maternal Crimes, Minor Calamities, and Occasional Moments of Grace,* women not only watch media stories of truly bad mothers with horror but also continually put themselves down as bad mothers with nobody's help.

8. The Jillian Johnson story (involving a woman whose baby died from accidental starvation), which was widely reported in 2017, comes to mind as a prime example. She breastfed with inadequate supply, reportedly "brainwashed" to abhor formula and to believe that the baby would get enough milk (according to a *USA Today* article posted online in March 2017).

9. For example, Barston 2012.

10. Ryan et al. 2013.

11. Grayson 2016:278.

12. Stuebe 2014.

13. Rich 1976.

14. Rothman [1989] 2000.

15. Rothman [1989] 2000.

16. Eckhardt and Hendershot 1984.

17. See Bobel 2001.

18. CDC 2016.

19. Jacqueline H. Wolf 2001.

20. Leavitt 1980.

21. Jacqueline H. Wolf 2001.

22. For example, Firestone 1970.

23. Nathoo and Ostry 2010.

24. Mills 1959.

25. Rothman 1989.

26. Hochschild 2013.

27. Rothman 2016:51.

28. Hays 1998.

29. Lareau 2003.

30. Hochschild 1989.

31. Tomori 2014.

32. Hays 1998; Damaske 2011.

33. Damaske 2011.

34. Reich 2010:169.

35. Reich 2016.

36. Barston 2012; Faircloth 2013; Jung 2015; Tuteur 2016a; Joan B. Wolf 2011.

37. Hays 1998.

38. Hays 1998.

39. Copelton et al. 2010.

40. Reich 2010.

41. Ginsburg and Rapp 1995; see also Angela Y. Davis 1981.

42. Devin uses gender-neutral they/their/them pronouns to refer to themself.

43. Allers 2017.

44. Grayson 2016.

45. Joan B. Wolf 2011.

46. Office of Minority Health. U.S. Department of Health and Human Services. https://minorityhealth.hhs.gov/omh/browse.aspx?lvl=3&lvlid=8. This information has been removed from the site.

47. Baby Prints. n.d. This graphic was found through a Google image search for "breast-feeding poster." The poster lists several benefits of breastfeeding and reads, "Extended breast feeding campaign by Baby Prints."

48. Blum 1999; Joan B. Wolf 2011; Copelton et al. 2010.

49. CDC 2014.

50. Jacqueline H. Wolf 2001.

51. Crenshaw 1989.

52. Grayson 2016; Jung 2015; Lepore 2013.

53. Merewood et al. 2005.

54. hooks 2000; Collins 1990.

55. I include Dr. Ameena Ali's name here to give her due credit for her ideas and for her organizational efforts with Chocolät Milk (a milk sharing collective). Accustomed to speaking with reporters, she treated our interview as an on-the-record conversation with her as an expert source. We did not discuss her personal experiences with breastfeeding.

56. Combined, the Facebook groups have millions of "likes." Breastfeeding Mama Talk alone garnered nearly a million (931,996) by mid-2017.

57. I analyzed posts from these three sites on four dates in 2016: April 20, June 19, September 6, and November 16.

58. My status as a researcher proved less interesting to some of the protestors who wished to speak with reporters instead, for the obvious reason that they wanted their voices amplified to make an immediate difference in the situation.

59. Haraway 1988.

60. Stacey 1988.

61. See Gamson (2015) for a discussion about his experience as a sociologist telling others' family stories; whenever he shared his writing with them, they inevitably changed the details and sometimes even the narrative.

62. Fabien 2017.

63. Welter 1966.

64. Barad 2003; Haraway 2016; Asberg et al. 2015.

65. A Google image search of this slogan will turn up several of these posters.

66. Latour 2005.

67. Barad's (2007) "intra-action" conveys the idea that individual phenomena (and individuals) emerge from their relations.

68. Simonds 2002.

69. Bartlett 2010.

70. Rothman 2016:26.

71. Dettwyler 1995.

72. Ryan et al. 2013.

73. Viveiros de Castro 2013. Please note that the term *natives* is inappropriate in American anthropology.

74. Barston 2012; Faircloth 2013; Jung 2015; Tuteur 2016a; Joan B. Wolf 2011.

75. Tsing 2005.

76. Hinde 2016.

77. Grayson 2016:276.

78. Said 1978.

79. Grayson 2016.

80. Grayson 2016.

81. Anthropologist Maia Boswell-Penc (2006) worries that feminists sometimes avoid breastfeeding controversies—such as the presence of toxins in the milk—because they are overly concerned that focusing on women's bodies only further essentializes them.

82. For example, Gmelch 1971.

83. See Rothman [1989] 2000 for an important discussion about the mothering experience as a process rather than a series of singular events.

84. Joan B. Wolf 2011.

85. Dykes 2006.

86. Plummer 2003; Smyth 2008.

87. Nussbaum 2011.

88. Reich 2016.

89. See the United States Breastfeeding Committee's website: http://www.usbreast feeding.org/.

90. Wall 2001.
91. For example, Jung 2015.
92. Marshall et al. 2007.
93. For example, Raju 2011.
94. Susan Falls (2017:93) wonders if the modifier *informal* might imply illegitimacy in contrast to milk banks, which presumably represent "formal" milk sharing.
95. Tomori 2014.
96. See Tomori 2014.
97. Conrad 1985, 2007; Rothman [1989] 2000.
98. Kleinman 1988.
99. Conrad 2007.
100. Policies might exclude "gay men" and fail to exclude men who have sex with men, who may not identify as gay.
101. Klugman 2010.
102. Carroll 2014.
103. Baby-Friendly USA 2012.
104. Tuteur 2016b.
105. Lording 2012.
106. For example, Mamo and Fosket 2009; Simonds et al. 2007.
107. See Foucault 1975.
108. Apple 1995.
109. Joan B. Wolf 2011.
110. Falls 2017:87.
111. Flaherman et al. 2012.
112. Tsing 2005.
113. Mayo Clinic 2018.
114. Crenshaw 1989.
115. In the wake of the 2017 Women's March, *intersectionality* became a popular concept people used to mean "diversity" or "multicultural" in an "add race and stir" manner not unlike tokenism. If Twitter discourse is any indication, the Trump-era alt-right brutalizes the concept, wielding it as an epithet against those whom they see as "liberal elites."
116. Roberts 1997.
117. Fraser 1998.
118. Currie 2013.
119. Barad 2003; Weasel 2016.
120. Allers 2017.
121. Collins 1990.
122. Gaskin 2009.
123. Mauthner 2016.
124. Butler 1990, 1993.
125. West and Zimmerman 1987.
126. Seidman 1995.
127. Drawn from Haraway 2016.
128. Collins 1990.

CHAPTER 2   CLEAVAGES

1. Hochschild 2013.
2. CDC 2016.
3. See Merewood et al. 2005.
4. CDC 2016.
5. For reviews of this medical and public health literature, see Whalen and Cramton 2010; U.S. Department of Health and Human Services 2011.
6. Schmied and Lupton 2001.
7. Joan B. Wolf 2011.
8. Reich 2011.
9. Reich 2011.
10. See Bartle 2010:123.
11. Blum 1999.
12. Pineau 2011.
13. Berry and Gribble 2008.
14. Stearns 2010.
15. The prime side effect of this drug, originally developed for stomach ailments (one brand is called "Vomit Stop"), is lactation, though some breastfeeders complain of weight gain. It is not a moneymaker for pharmaceutical companies, and some think this is the reason it is not approved for lactation. Reglan remains legal even though it affects hormones and may cause confusion, moodiness, and blurred vision. Many doctors refuse to prescribe Reglan because it is not worth the ill effects.
16. For example, Dennis 1999; McCarter-Spaulding and Kearney 2001.
17. Dewey (1998; cf. Kramer et al. 2002) conducted a large study that contradicted the conventional idea that formula-fed babies gain weight faster.
18. Dewey 2001.
19. Flaherman et al. 2012.
20. Lepore 2013.
21. See Stuart-Macadam and Dettwyler 1995 for a biocultural perspective on this controversy.
22. Quandt 1995.
23. Halley 2007.
24. Scrinis 2013.
25. For example, Lucas and Cole 1990; Lanting et al. 1994.
26. Fewtrell 2004.
27. Two trade books outline competing interpretations of the data: *Lactivism: How Feminists and Fundamentalists, Hippies and Yuppies, and Physicians and Politicians Made Breastfeeding Big Business and Bad Policy* by Courtney Jung (2015) and *The Big Letdown: How Medicine, Big Business, and Feminism Undermine Breastfeeding* by Kimberly Seals Allers (2017). Jung questions the science that supports breastfeeding as preventive medicine. She assumes that women feel undue pressure to breastfeed as they respond to thin scientific evidence that overinflates the value of breast milk. Taking the opposite position, Allers digs into shortcomings of scientific investigations, noting that they are

stacked against showing breastfeeding's true range of benefits. She argues that the milk is probably even more valuable than we think and claims that outside interests (like formula companies) limit the research into the subject. (Allers also extols the act of suckling, not just the good chemistry of breast milk.) Also, see Grayson 2016.

28. See Hinde, n.d.; see also Hinde 2016.

29. This trend among bodybuilders and other high performance athletes is not well documented, but it makes for good clickbait. See Easter 2015.

30. Supposedly fast twitch muscle fibers make for an athlete with more speed and agility and slow twitch muscle fibers support physical endurance.

31. HIV can be transmitted through breast milk; research suggests a 14 percent chance of transmission in the absence of retroviral drugs (Zeigler et al. 1985). Also note that in places where water is contaminated, breastfeeding prevents infant deaths more than it poses a risk of HIV transmission (Van Esterik 2010).

32. Bar-Yam 2010:106.

33. Bar-Yam 2010:106.

34. To flash pasteurize, barely bring the glass-bottled milk to a boil and then immediately immerse it in freezing water.

35. One frequently cited study (Mennella et al. 2001) involved an experiment with some women drinking carrot juice during late pregnancy and early breastfeeding. Researchers later evaluated the weaned children's expressions when they first tasted carrots. It seemed that the babies more familiar with the taste looked happier about that first spoonful. Even though the observers rated their facial expressions on a scale from one to nine, it still seems a ripe opportunity for confirmation basis—seeing the results that one expects to see. This is not to say that tastes do not transfer, just that the science on the question remains limited.

36. Shim et al. 2011.

37. Keim et al. 2013.

38. Healy 2013; see Carter and Foster 2016 for a discussion of the themes in these sorts of news pieces.

39. Palmquist and Doehler 2014, 2016; Reyes-Foster et al. 2015, Carter et al. 2015.

40. Reyes-Foster et al. 2015.

41. Hanson and Korotkova 2002.

42. Hassiotou et al. 2013, Raju 2011.

43. Saha et al. 2015.

44. Hill and Reed 2013.

45. Allers 2017.

46. Wiley 2016.

47. U.S. National Library of Medicine 2018.

48. Grayson 2016.

49. Li 2014.

50. Alexander 1981; Kleinman 1988.

CHAPTER 3   THE MOTHER OF INVENTION

1. Ryan, Bissell, and Alexander 2010.
2. Waltz 2014.
3. The irony that any and all divergence from the perceived norm could be "exceptional" is not lost on me. It reminds me of how Americans like to be unique, just like everybody else. In obstetric medicine, so many pregnant women receive the high risk label that the designation loses its original meaning (Rothman 2007).
4. Park 2006.
5. Gribble 2006.
6. Reich 2010.
7. Reich 2010.
8. "I did then what I knew how to do. Now that I know better, I do better." Maya Angelou to Oprah Winfrey, as reported by Winfrey on October 19, 2011, "The Powerful Lesson Maya Angelou Taught Oprah," Oprah's Lifeclass (website), http://www.oprah.com/oprahs-lifeclass/the-powerful-lesson-maya-angelou-taught-oprah-video.
9. Gribble 2007a.
10. American Academy of Pediatrics 2012.
11. Allers 2017; Bartick et al. 2016.
12. Halley 2007.
13. Giles 2010.
14. Giles 2010.
15. Dykes 2006.
16. Dykes 2006.
17. Stearns 2010.
18. Rothman 2016:9.
19. Layne 1999.
20. Rothman 2016.
21. See Haraway 1985.
22. Bartlett 2010.
23. Hays 1998.
24. Rothman [1989] 2000.
25. Oparah and Bonaparte 2015.
26. Reich 2011.
27. See Rothman 2016 for a comparison of the food and birth movements.
28. Gribble 2010:72.
29. Gribble 2007b, 2010.
30. Ryan, Todres, and Alexander 2010.
31. Rothman [1989] 2000.

CHAPTER 4   MILKING THE SYSTEM

1. Falls 2017:158.
2. Falls 2017:202.

3. Nearly a third of the eighty-three interview respondents worked in the birth or breastfeeding fields—some as volunteers or lay experts (n=15) and some as professionals (n=12).

4. Roxanne gave birth alone without her husband's or a midwife's assistance.

5. Allers 2012.

6. Allers 2017.

7. Hartman 2007.

8. For example, Jung 2015; Tuteur 2016a.

9. Falls 2017:23.

10. There are no quantitative data on "exceptional breastfeeding" as a category. The public hears the advice to "exclusive[ly] breastfeed for six months and continue to breastfeed until one year" as the bounded norm. Everything else seems exceptional in some way.

11. Both had just finished their service with U.S. military.

12. Faircloth 2009.

13. Joan B. Wolf 2011.

14. Bartle 2010:125.

15. Rapp 2000.

16. See Hausman 2010 for a discussion on breastfeeding and risk.

17. I later discovered that social workers surreptitiously evaluate the parenting fitness of prospective foster parents when they attend the mandatory training sessions. Had I known, I may not have ventured to ask about breastfeeding.

18. Benjamin 2016.

19. Foucault 1973.

20. Auerbach 1987.

21. Weston A. Price Foundation 2018.

22. Allers 2017.

23. Carroll and Reiger 2005.

24. Torres 2014.

25. Bobel 2002.

26. See http://acquandastanford.com/ for links.

27. MacDonald et al. 2016.

28. Tomori et al. 2016.

29. Tomori et al. 2016.

30. The stigmatized breastfeeders studied by Tomori et al. (2016:178) suffered social isolation as a result of their "avoidance of health professionals and others who might judge them."

31. Rothman 2007.

32. Kukla 2006.

33. Davis 2017.

34. According to salary.com and payscale.com, the national average annual incomes are as follows: nurse midwives, $96,970; hospital-based lactation consultants, $77,297; and direct-entry midwives, $60,000. The reported averages for birth doulas ranged widely from $29,000 to $50,000.

35. See Bartle 2010:128–129 for a discussion on breast milk and authoritative knowledge in neonatal units.

36. Bartle 2010.

37. Cassidy and El-Tom 2010.

38. Bartle 2010.

39. Joan B. Wolf 2011.

40. Kukla 2006.

41. U.S. Department of Health and Human Services 2011.

42. Galtry 2003.

43. Murtagh and Moulton 2011.

44. See Bartlett 2010 for how modern understandings of time interfere with the breastfeeding experience.

45. Breastfeeding in Combat Boots, n.d.

46. Allers 2017:136–138.

47. Allers 2017:131.

48. Rothman 2016:11–12 notes that middle-class women have a tendency "to take pregnancy . . . as a big reading assignment."

49. Falls 2017:150.

50. Benjamin 2016.

51. Benjamin 2013.

52. Althusser 1967.

53. Bourdieu 1979.

54. A February 25, 2011, story on NPR, "Breast Milk Ice Cream A Hit At London Store," by Bill Chappell highlighted this apparently popular choice at a store in London (http://www.npr.org/sections/thetwo-way/2011/02/25/134056923/breast-milk-ice-cream-a-hit-at-london-store).

55. Rothman 2016.

56. Gaskin 2003, 2009.

57. After speaking at a Birth Round Up event in Texas, Gaskin came under fire for seeming to dismiss racism in birth outcomes. The comments sections of several birth-related internet groups lit up, and more than one anti-Gaskin petition circulated. She apologized. See Griffin 2017.

58. According to 2015 CDC reports, infant mortality for black babies is 11.11 per 1,000 live births, whereas for whites, it is 5.06. The maternal mortality rate is on the rise among all groups in the United States, while they are declining in other parts of the world (Murray et al. 2016). Black woman are three to four times more likely to die from pregnancy or birth-related complications than white women (MacDorman et al. 2017). According to the CDC's 2016 "Breastfeeding Report Card," 54 percent of black women initiate breastfeeding compared to 74 percent of whites, 80 percent of Hispanics, and 81 percent of Asians / Pacific Islanders.

59. Stanford 2016.

60. Blactavist (@Blactavist). 2016.

CHAPTER 5   BUSTING BINARIES

1. Laura Mamo also tangles with some of the tensions between normalizing and subverting procreative norms in her book *Queering Reproduction* (2007) about lesbian family building.
2. Franz Boas brought the concept from German philosophy to his anthropology students at Columbia University in the early twentieth century.
3. Campo 2010.
4. Rothman [1989] 2000.
5. Several of the breastfeeders I talked to disbelieved the notion that pregnancy and aging, not breastfeeding, cause the changes in breast shape and elasticity.
6. Epstein-Gilboa 2010; Giles 2003.
7. Milky Way Foundation, n.d.
8. Inspired by the Katie Hinde's blog. See Hinde, n.d.
9. Breakey et al. 2015.
10. Bartol and Bagnell 2014.
11. Rey et al. 2013.
12. http://mammalssuck.blogspot.com.
13. Salamon 2010.
14. Svanborg et al. 2003.
15. For example, Vohr et al. 2006.
16. Benjamin 2013.
17. Falls 2017.

CHAPTER 6   FLUIDITY OF THE FAMILY

1. Franklin 2013.
2. Fildes 1988.
3. Konrad 2005.
4. Emile Durkheim (1897) offers the term *anomie* to describe the isolated existence most people experience as part of capitalism.
5. Tomori et al. 2016.
6. Granovetter 1973.
7. Brill 2001.
8. Mehra and Bishop 2004.
9. Lev et al. 2008.
10. Falls 2017:79.
11. This context highlights the limits of the word *recipient,* which is dehumanizing and passive sounding. Someone who obtains sperm from a sperm bank takes action to become a parent. Caregivers who receive milk donations are also actively performing care, not passively accepting food for their babies.
12. These conservative maneuvers include the now-defunct Defense of Marriage Act and antigay adoption laws, which continue to be proposed in state legislatures.
13. Collins 1990.

14. Rothman [1989] 2000.

15. For example, Naples 2004; Sheff 2013.

16. McKenna and Gettler 2015.

17. The influential American Academy of Pediatrics insists that cosleeping is danger-ous. Anthropologists tend not to agree, in part because the practice is ancient and prac-ticed all over the world. McKenna usually advocates breastsleeping with the caveat that parents should not be under the influence of alcohol or other sedative drugs, which make it more likely that they could accidentally roll over and smother their infant. The lactation consultants I observed suggested minimal bed coverings and only sleeping on mattresses (versus plush sofas) as additional protection from suffocation.

18. Zizzo 2009.

19. Ryan, Todres, and Alexander 2010.

CHAPTER 7   "OUTPOURING OF SUPPORT"

1. Falls 2017:155.

2. Falls 2017:130.

3. Locklin and Naber 1993.

4. Specific details about the group and poster have not been provided to preserve anonymity.

5. Tongue-ties and lip-ties happen when the strip of skin under the tongue or in front of the lip is shorter than usual, a condition thought to hinder a comfortable mouth-to-nipple latch. Minor surgery (or cutting with a fingernail, as some midwives will do) can detach the skin.

6. Reich 2016:214.

7. Seen on a car's bumper sticker.

8. LeMieux 2016.

9. Reich 2016.

10. Goffman 1956.

11. Gribble and Hausman 2012; Gribble 2012; Carter and Foster 2016.

12. Palmquist and Doehler 2016; Palmquist and Doehler 2014; Reyes-Foster et al. 2015.

13. Jacqueline H. Wolf 2001.

14. Pineau 2012.

15. Grayson 2016:213.

16. Shaw 2007.

17. It is similar to Charis M. Cussins's (1998) finding that surrogates varied in their kin-like status depending on how transparent or opaque their arrangement was.

18. This website has a bad reputation in the milk-sharing community because of these sorts of interactions, because the site itself is a money-making venture and the milk is sold, and because babies are not the only ones to get the milk.

19. Hausman 2010.

20. See Shaw and Webb 2015.

21. Bodybuilders and fetishists in the market for breast milk need not apply.

22. For an example, see Post Bedtime Creations' shop at http://www.postbedtime creations.com.

23. A *Reply All* podcast titled "Milk Wanted" traces one mother's frustrating attempts to find enough milk for her formula-averse infant. See episode 57, March 9, 2016, https://gimletmedia.com/episode/57-milk-wanted/.

24. Azema and Callahan 2003.

25. Palmquist and Doehler 2016; Palmquist and Doehler 2014; Reyes-Foster et al. 2015.

26. Cambodia banned Ambrosia from these exports in March 2017.

27. I did not interview anyone who sold her milk. I received no response to messages I sent to people who posted milk for sale on onlythebreast.com. In comments sections of various breastfeeding sites online, I observed self-described milk sellers and potential milk sellers complain about the unofficial moratorium on selling milk among their peers.

28. See Shaw 2010 for a discussion on the ethics of milk sharing.

29. Giles 2003.

30. Medolac, n.d.

31. Plummer 2003.

32. Ryan, Bissell, and Alexander 2010.

33. Rudrappa 2015.

34. Cassidy 2012.

REFERENCES

Alexander, Linda. 1981. "The Double-Bind between Dialysis Patients and Their Health Practitioners." In *The Relevance of Social Sciences for Medicine*, edited by L. Eisenberg and Arthur Kleinman, 307–309. Dordrecht, Holland: D. Reidel.

Allers, Kimberly Seals. 2012. "Breastfeeding: Some Slavery Crap?" *Ebony Magazine*, August 31, 2012. http://www.ebony.com/wellness-empowerment/breastfeeding -some-slavery-crap#axzz4RQDJjMwo.

———. 2017. *The Big Letdown: How Medicine, Big Business, and Feminism Undermine Breastfeeding*. New York: St. Martin's Press.

Althusser, Louis. 1967. *Contradiction and Over-Determination*. London: New Left Review.

American Academy of Pediatrics. 2012. "Policy on Breastfeeding and Human Milk." Accessed May 23, 2018. http://www2.aap.org/breastfeeding/files/pdf/breast feeding2012execsum.pdf.

Apple, Rima D. 1995. "Constructing Mothers: Scientific Motherhood in the Nineteenth and Twentieth Centuries." *Social History of Medicine* 8 (2): 161–178.

Asberg, Cecilia, Kathrin Thiele, and Iris Van Der Tuin. 2015. "Speculative *Before* the Turn: Reintroducing Feminist Materialist Performativity." *Cultural Studies Review* 21 (2): 145–172.

Auerbach, K. G., and L. M. Gartner. 1987. "Breastfeeding and Human Milk: Their Association with Jaundice in the Neonate." *Clinics in Perinatology* 14 (1): 89–107.

Azema, Emilie, and Stacey Callahan. 2003. "Breast Milk Donors in France: A Portrait of the Typical Donor and the Utility of Milk Banking in the French Breastfeeding Context." *Journal of Human Lactation* 19 (2): 199–202.

Baby-Friendly USA. 2012. "Ten Steps and International Code." Accessed May 23, 2018. https://www.babyfriendlyusa.org/about-us/10-steps-and-international-code.

Baby Prints. n.d. "His Well Being Depends on You." Accessed May 30, 2018. https:// i.pinimg.com/236x/b1/9c/88/b19c886ea6b823742b3e3051c6435f0e--midwife -training-toddler-nutrition.jpg.

Barad, Karen. 2003. "Posthumanist Performativity: Toward an Understanding of How Matter Comes to Matter." *Signs* 28 (3): 801–831.

———. 2007. *Meeting the Universe Halfway: Quantum Physics and the Entanglement of Matter and Meaning*. Durham: Duke University Press.

Barston, Suzanne. 2012. *Bottled Up: How the Way We Feed Babies Has Come to Define Motherhood and Why It Shouldn't*. Berkeley: University of California Press.

Bartick, M. C., E. B. Schwarz, B. D. Green, B. J. Jegier, A. G. Reinhold, T. T. Colaizy, D. L. Bogen, A. J. Schaefer, and A. M. Stuebe. 2016. "Suboptimal Breastfeeding in the United States: Maternal and Pediatric Health Outcomes and Costs." *Maternal and Child Nutrition* 13 (1).

Bartle, Carol. 2010. "Going with the Flow: Contemporary Discourses of Donor Breast-milk Use in a Neonatal Intensive Care Setting." In *Giving Breastmilk: Body Ethics and Contemporary Breastfeeding Practice*, edited by Rhonda Shaw and Alison Bartlett, 122–133. Bradford, Ontario: Demeter Press.

Bartlett, Alison. 2010. "Breastfeeding and Time: In Search of a Language for Pleasure and Agency." In *Giving Breastmilk: Body Ethics and Contemporary Breastfeeding Practice*, edited by Rhonda Shaw and Alison Bartlett, 222–235. Bradford, Ontario: Demeter Press.

Bartol, Frank F., and Carol A. Bagnell. 2014. "Lactocrine Programming of Postnatal Reproductive Tract Development." Presented at the American Dairy Science Asso-ciation, American Society of Animal Science, and Canadian Society of Animal Sci-ence joint annual meeting in Kansas City, Missouri, July 20–24, 2014.

Bar-Yam, Naomi Bromberg. 2010. "The Story of the Mothers' Milk Bank of New England." In *Giving Breastmilk: Body Ethics and Contemporary Breastfeeding Practice*, edited by Rhonda Shaw and Alison Bartlett, 98–109. Bradford, Ontario: Demeter Press.

Benjamin, Ruha. 2013. *People's Science: Bodies and Rights on the Stem Cell Frontier*. Palo Alto: Stanford University Press.

———. 2016. "Informed Refusal: Toward a Justice-Based Bioethics." *Science, Tech-nology, and Human Values*. 41 (6): 967–990. http://www.ruhabenjamin.com/a/wp-content/uploads/2016/06/2016-Informed-Refusal.pdf.

Berry, Nina J., and Karleen D. Gribble. 2008. "Breast Is No Longer Best: Promoting Normal Infant Feeding." *Maternal and Child Nutrition* 4 (1): 74–79.

Blactavist (@Blactavist). 2016. "Purposely take back OUR power!! Our milk is revolu-tionary. #nia #kwanzaa." December 30, 2016. instagram.com/p/BOqXbFohGQK/.

Blum, Linda. 1999. *At the Breast: Ideologies of Breastfeeding and Motherhood in the Con-temporary United States*. Boston: Beacon Press.

Bobel, Chris. 2001. "Bounded Liberation: A Focused Study of La Leche League Inter-national." *Gender and Society* 15 (1): 130–151.

———. 2002. *The Paradox of Natural Mothering*. Philadelphia: Temple University Press.

Boswell-Penc, Maia. 2006. *Tainted Milk: Breastmilk, Feminisms, and the Politics of Envi-ronmental Degradation*. Albany: State University of New York Press.

Bourdieu, Pierre. 1979. *Distinction: A Social Critique of the Judgment of Taste*. Cambridge, Mass.: Harvard University Press.

Breakey, A., K. Hinde, C. R. Valeggia, A. Sinofsky, and P. T. Ellison. 2015. "Illness in Breastfeeding Infants Relates to Concentration of Lactoferrin and Secretory Immu-noglobulin A in Mother's Milk." *Evolution, Medicine, and Public Health* 1:21–31.

Breastfeeding in Combat Boots. n.d. "Home Page." Accessed December 1, 2016. http://breastfeedingincombatboots.com/.

Brill, Stephanie. 2001. *The Essential Guide to Lesbian Conception, Pregnancy, and Birth*. New York: Alyson Books.

Butler, Judith. 1990. *Gender Trouble: Feminism and the Subversion of Gender*. New York: Routledge.

———. 1993. *Bodies That Matter: On the Discourse Limits of Sex*. New York: Routledge.

Campo, Monica. 2010. "The Lactating Body and Conflicting Ideals of Sexuality, Motherhood and Self." *Giving Breastmilk: Body Ethics and Contemporary Breastfeeding Practice*, edited by Rhonda Shaw and Alison Bartlett, 51–63. Bradford, Ontario: Demeter Press.

Carroll, Katherine. 2014. "Body Dirt or Liquid Gold? How the 'Safety' for Use of Donated Breastmilk Is Constructed in Neonatal Intensive Care." *Social Studies of Science* 44 (3): 466–485.

———. 2015. "Breastmilk Donation as Care Work." In *Ethnographies of Breastfeeding: Cultural Contexts and Confrontations*, edited by Tanya Cassidy and Abdullahi El Tom, 173–186. London: Bloomsbury.

Carroll, Katherine, and Kerreen Reiger. 2005. "Fluid Experts: Lactation Experts as Postmodern Professional Specialists." *Health Sociology Review* 14 (2): 101–110.

Carter, Shannon K., and Beatriz Reyes-Foster. 2016. "Pure Gold for Broken Bodies: Discursive Techniques Constructing Milk Banking and Peer Milk Sharing in U.S. News." *Symbolic Interaction* 39 (3): 353–373.

Carter, Shannon K., Beatriz Reyes-Foster, and Tiffany L. Rogers. 2015. "Liquid Gold or Russian Roulette?" *Health, Risk, and Society* 17 (1): 30–45.

Cassidy, Tanya M. 2012. "Making Milky Matches: Globalization, Maternal Trust, and 'Lactivist' Online Networking." *Journal of the Motherhood Initiative* 3 (1): 226–240.

Cassidy, Tanya M., and Abdullahi El-Tom. 2010. "Comparing Sharing and Banking Milk: Issues of Gift Exchange and Community in the Sudan and Ireland." In *Giving Breastmilk: Body Ethics and Contemporary Breastfeeding Practice*, edited by Rhonda Shaw and Alison Bartlett, 110–121. Bradford, Ontario: Demeter Press.

Centers for Disease Control and Prevention (CDC). 2014. "Breastfeeding Report Card." Accessed January 15, 2017. https://www.cdc.gov/breastfeeding/data/reportcard.htm.

———. 2015. "Breastfeeding Report Card." Accessed May 23, 2018. https://www.cdc .gov/breastfeeding/data/reportcard.htm.

———. 2016. "Breastfeeding Report Card." Accessed January 15, 2017. https://www .cdc.gov/breastfeeding/data/reportcard.htm.

Collins, Patricia Hill. 1990. *Black Feminist Thought: Knowledge, Consciousness, and the Politics of Empowerment*. New York: Routledge.

Conrad, Peter. 1985. "The Meaning of Medications: Another Look at Compliance." *Social Science and Medicine* 20 (1): 29–37.

———. 2007. *The Medicalization of Society: On the Transformation of Human Conditions into Treatable Disorders*. Baltimore: Johns Hopkins University Press.

Copelton, Denise A., Rebecca McGee, Andrew Coco, Isis Shanbaky, and Timothy Riley. 2010. "The Ideological Work of Infant Feeding." In *Giving Breastmilk: Body Ethics and Contemporary Breastfeeding Practice*, edited by Rhonda Shaw and Alison Bartlett, 24–38. Bradford, Ontario: Demeter Press.

Crenshaw, Kimberle. 1989. "Demarginalizing the Intersection of Race and Sex: A Black Feminist Critique of Antidiscrimination Doctrine, Feminist Theory and Antiracist Politics." *University of Chicago Legal Forum*: 139.

Currie, Donya. 2013. "Breastfeeding Rates for Black US Women Increase, but Lag Overall: Continuing Disparity Raises Concerns." *Nation's Health* 43 (3): 1–20. http://thenationshealth.aphapublications.org/content/43/3/1.3.

Cussins, Charis M. 1998. *Cyborg Babies: From Techno-Sex to Techno-Tots*, edited by Robbie Davis-Floyd and Joseph Dumit, 40–66. New York: Routledge.

Damaske, Sarah. 2011. *For the Family? How Class and Gender Shape Women's Work.* Oxford: Oxford University Press.

Davis, Angela Y. 1981. *Women, Race, and Class.* New York: Vintage Books.

Davis, Dana-Ain. 2017. "Race, Prematurity, and Birthing Justice." Presented at the Spring Conference of the American Ethnological Society, Stanford, California, April 1, 2017.

Dennis, C. L. 1999. "Theoretical Underpinnings of Breastfeeding Confidence: A Self-Efficacy Framework." *Journal of Human Lactation* 15 (3): 195–201.

Dettwyler, Katherine A. 1995. "Beauty and the Breast: The Cultural Context of Breastfeeding in the United States." In *Biocultural Perspectives on Breastfeeding*, edited by Patricia Stuart-Macadam and Katherine A. Dettwyler, 167–216. New York: Aldine de Gruyter.

Dewey, K. G. 1998. "Growth Characteristics of Breast-Fed Compared to Formula-Fed Infants." *Neonatology* 74 (2): 94–105.

———. 2001. "Maternal and Fetal Stress Are Associated with Impaired Lactogenesis in Humans." *Journal of Nutrition* 131 (11): 3012–3015.

Durkheim, Emile. (1897) 1951. *Suicide: A Study in Sociology.* Translated by John A. Spaulding and George Simpson. Glencoe: Free Press.

Dykes, Fiona. 2006. *Breastfeeding in Hospital: Mothers, Midwives and the Production Line.* New York: Routledge.

Easter, Michael. 2015. "Bodybuilders Are Drinking Human Breast Milk. Are They Insane, or Super Insane?" *Men's Health*, February 19, 2015. https://www.menshealth.com/fitness/a19530877/human-breast-milk-and-bodybuilding/.

Eckhardt, K. W., and G. E. Hendershot. 1984. "Analysis of the Reversal in Breastfeeding Trends in the Early 1970s." *Public Health Reports* 99:410–415.

Epstein-Gilboa, Keren. 2010. "Breastfeeding Envy: Unresolved Patriarchal Envy and the Obstruction of Physiologically-Based Nursing Patterns." In *Giving Breastmilk: Body Ethics and Contemporary Breastfeeding Practice*, edited by Rhonda Shaw and Alison Bartlett, 205–221. Bradford, Ontario: Demeter Press.

Fabien, Vanessa. 2017. "My Body, My Pain: Listen to Me and All Black Women." *The Root*, April 16, 2017. http://www.theroot.com/my-body-my-pain-listen-to-me-and-all-black-women-1794332651.

Faircloth, Charlotte. 2009. "Mothering as Identity-Work: Long-Term Breastfeeding and Intensive Motherhood." *Anthropology News* 50 (2): 15–17.

———. 2013. *Militant Lactivism? Attachment Parenting and Intensive Motherhood in the UK and France.* New York: Berghahn Books.

Falls, Susan. 2017. *White Gold: Stories of Breast Milk Sharing.* Lincoln: University of Nebraska Press.

Fewtrell, M. S. 2004. "The Long-Term Benefits of Having Been Breast-Fed." *Current Paediatrics* 14 (2): 97–103.

Fildes, Valerie. 1988. *Wet Nursing: A History from Antiquity to Present*. New York: Basil and Blackwell.

Firestone, Shulamith. 1970. *The Dialectic of Sex*. New York: Farrar, Strauss, and Giroux.

Flaherman, Valerie J., Katherine G. Hicks, Michael D. Cabana, and Kathryn A. Lee. 2012. "Maternal Experience of Interactions with Providers among Mothers with Milk Supply Concern." *Clinical Pediatrics* 51 (8): 778–784.

Foucault, Michel. 1973. *The Birth of the Clinic: An Archaeology of Medical Perception*. New York: Vintage Books.

———. 1975. *Discipline and Punish: The Birth of the Prison*. New York: Vintage Books.

Franklin, Sarah. 2013. *Biological Relatives: IVF, Stem Cells, and the Future of Kinship*. Durham: Duke University Press.

Fraser, Gertrude J. 1998. *African American Midwifery in the South: Dialogues of Birth, Race, and Memory*. Cambridge, Mass.: Harvard University Press.

Galtry, Judith. 2003. "The Impact on Breastfeeding of Labour Market Policy and Practice in Ireland, Sweden, and the USA." *Social Science and Medicine* 57 (1): 167–177.

Gamson, Joshua. 2015. *Modern Families: Stories of Extraordinary Journeys to Kinship*. New York: New York University Press.

Gaskin, Ina May. 2003. *Ina May's Guide to Childbirth*. New York: Bantam Books.

———. 2009. *Ina May's Guide to Breastfeeding*. New York: Bantam Books.

Giles, Fiona. 2003. *Fresh Milk: The Secret Lives of Breasts*. New York: Simon and Schuster.

———. 2010. "From 'Gift of Loss' to Self Care: The Significance of Induced Lactation in Takashi Miike's *Visitor Q*." In *Giving Breastmilk: Body Ethics and Contemporary Breastfeeding Practice*, edited by Rhonda Shaw and Alison Bartlett, 236–250. Bradford, Ontario: Demeter Press.

Ginsburg, Faye, and Rayna Rapp, eds. 1995. *Conceiving the New World Order: The Global Politics of Reproduction*. Berkeley: University of California Press.

Gmelch, George. 1971. "Baseball Magic." *Society* 8 (8): 39–41.

Goffman, Erving. 1956. "The Presentation of Self in Everyday Life." New York: Random House.

Granovetter, Mark S. 1973. "The Strength of Weak Ties." *American Journal of Sociology* 78 (6): 1360–1380.

Grayson, Jennifer. 2016. *Unlatched: The Evolution of Breastfeeding and the Making of a Controversy*. New York: HarperCollins.

Gribble, Karleen. 2006. "Mental Health, Attachment and Breastfeeding: Implications for Adopted Children and Their Mothers." *International Breastfeeding Journal* 1 (5). https://internationalbreastfeedingjournal.biomedcentral.com/articles/10.1186/1746-4358-1-5.

———. 2007a. "A Model for Caregiving of Adopted Children after Institutionalization." *Journal of Child and Adolescent Psychiatric Nursing* 20 (1): 14–26.

———. 2007b. "'As Good as Chocolate' and 'Better than Ice Cream': How Toddler, and Older, Breastfeeders Experience Breastfeeding." *Early Child Development and Care* 8:1067–1082.

———. 2010. "Receiving and Enjoying Milk: What Breastfeeding Means to Children." In *Giving Breastmilk: Body Ethics and Contemporary Breastfeeding Practice*, edited by Rhonda Shaw and Alison Bartlett, 64–82. Bradford, Ontario: Demeter Press.

———. 2012. "Biomedical Ethics and Peer-to-Peer Milk Sharing." *Clinical Lactation* 3 (3): 108–114.

Gribble, Karleen D., and Bernice L. Hausman. 2012. "Milk Sharing and Formula Feeding: Infant Feeding Risks in Comparative Perspective." *Australasian Medical Journal* 5 (5): 275–283.

Griffin, Samantha. 2017. "The Ina May Gaskin Racial Gaffe Heard 'round the Midwifery World." *Rewire News*, April 26, 2017. https://rewire.news/article/2017/04/26/ina-may-gaskin-racial-gaffe-heard-round-midwifery-world/.

Halley, Jean O'Malley. 2007. *Boundaries of Touch: Parenting and Adult-Child Intimacy*. Urbana: University of Illinois Press.

Hanson, L. Å., and M. Korotkova. 2002. "The Role of Breastfeeding in Prevention of Neonatal Infection." *Seminars in Neonatology* 7 (4): 275–281.

Haraway, Donna J. 1985. "Manifesto for Cyborgs: Science, Technology, and Socialist Feminism in the 1980s." *Socialist Review* 80:65–108.

———. 1988. "Situated Knowledges: The Science Question in Feminism and the Privilege of Partial Perspective." *Feminist Studies* 14 (3): 575–599.

———. 2016. *Staying with the Trouble: Making Kin in the Chthulucene*. Durham: Duke University Press.

Hartman, Saidiya. 2007. *Lose Your Mother: A Journey along the Atlantic Slave Route*. New York: Farrar, Strauss, and Giroux.

Hassiotou, Foteini, Donna T. Geddes, and Peter E. Hartmann. 2013. "Cells in Human Milk: State of the Science." *Journal of Human Lactation* 29 (2): 171–182.

Hausman, Bernice L. 2010. "Risk and Culture Revisited: Breastfeeding and the 2002 West Nile Virus Scare in the United States." In *Giving Breastmilk: Body Ethics and Contemporary Breastfeeding Practice*, edited by Rhonda Shaw and Alison Bartlett, 175–190. Bradford, Ontario: Demeter Press.

Hays, Sharon. 1998. *The Cultural Contradictions of Motherhood*. New Haven: Yale University Press.

Healy, Michelle. 2013. "Buying Milk Online? It May Be Contaminated." *USA Today*, October 21, 2013. https://www.usatoday.com/story/news/nation/2013/10/21/breast-milk-bacteria/3002973/.

Hill, Meg, and Kathryn Reed. 2013. "Pregnancy, Breast-feeding, and Marijuana: A Review Article." *Obstetrical and Gynecological Survey* 68 (10): 710–718.

Hinde, Katie. 2016. "What We Don't Know about Mother's Milk." TEDWomen October 2016 video. Accessed March 28, 2017. https://www.ted.com/talks/katie_hinde_what_we_don_t_know_about_mother_s_milk.

———. n.d. *Mammals Suck* (blog). Accessed May 23, 2018. http://mammalssuck.blogspot.com/.

Hochschild, Arlie Russell. 2013. *The Outsourced Self: What Happens When We Pay Others to Live Our Lives for Us*. London: Picador.

Hochschild, Arlie Russell, with Anne Machung. 1989. *The Second Shift: Working Parents and the Revolution at Home*. New York: Viking/Penguin.

hooks, bell. 2000. *Feminist Theory: From Margin to Center*. 2nd ed. London: Pluto Press.

Jung, Courtney. 2015. *Lactivism: How Feminists and Fundamentalists, Hippies and Yuppies, and Physicians and Politicians Made Breastfeeding Big Business and Bad Policy*. New York: Basic Books.

Keim, Sarah A., Joseph S. Hogan, Kelly A. McNamara, Vishnu Gudimetla, Jesse J. Kwiek, and Sheela R. Geraghty. 2013. "Microbial Contamination of Human Milk Purchased via the Internet." *Pediatrics* 32 (5): 1227–1235.

Kleinman, Arthur. 1988. *The Illness Narratives: Suffering, Healing, and the Human Condition*. New York: Basic Books.

Klugman, Craig M. 2010. "Blood Donation and Its Metaphors." *American Journal of Bioethics* 10 (2): 46–47.

Konrad, Monica. 2005. *Nameless Relations: Anonymity, Melanesia and Reproductive Gift Exchange between British Ova Donors and Recipients*. New York: Berghahn Books.

Kramer, Michael S., Tong Guo, Robert W. Platt, Stanley Shapiro, Jean-Paul Collet, Beverley Chalmers, Ellen Hodnett, Zinaida Sevkovskaya, Irina Dzikovich, and Irina Vanilovich for the PROBIT Study Group. 2002. "Breastfeeding and Infant Growth: Biology or Bias?" *Pediatrics* 110 (2): 343–347.

Kukla, Rebecca. 2006. "Ethics and Ideology in Breastfeeding Advocacy Campaigns." *Hypatia* 21 (1): 157–180.

Lanting, C. I., M. Huisman, E. R. Boersma, B. C. L. Touwen, and V. Fidler. 1994. "Neurological Differences between 9-Year-Old Children Fed Breast-Milk or Formula-Milk as Babies." *Lancet* 344:1319–1322.

Lareau, Annette. 2003. *Unequal Childhoods: Class, Race, and Family Life*. Berkeley: University of California Press.

Latour, Bruno. 2005. *Reassembling the Social: An Introduction to Actor-Network Theory*. New York: Oxford University Press.

Layne, Linda. 1999. "I Remember the Day I Shopped for Your Layette: Consumer Goods, Fetuses, and Feminism in the Context of Pregnancy Loss." In *Fetal Subjects, Feminist Positions*, edited by Lynn M. Morgan and Meredith W. Michaels, 251–278. Philadelphia: University of Pennsylvania Press.

Leavitt, Judith Walzer. 1980. "Birthing and Anesthesia: The Debate over Twilight Sleep." *Signs* 6 (1): 147–164.

LeMieux, Julianna. 2016. "Fed Is Best: Great Message, Not So Great Science." *American Council on Health and Science*, October 5, 2016. http://www.acsh.org/news/2016/10/05/fed-best-great-message-not-so-great-science-10240.

Lepore, Jill. 2013. *The Mansion of Happiness: A History of Life and Death*. New York: Vintage Books.

Lev, Arlene Istar, Gwendolyn Dean, Lauren Difilippis, Kim Evernham, Larin McLaughlin, and Cynthia Phillips. 2008. "Dykes and Tykes: A Virtual Lesbian Community." *Journal of Lesbian Studies* 9 (1–2): 81–94.

Li, Jialin Camille. 2014. "Formula Feeding and the Social Body: Exploring the Bodies in Infant Feeding in Contemporary China." Paper presented at the annual meeting of the American Sociological Association, San Francisco, California, August 16, 2014.

Locklin, M. P., and S. J. Naber. 1993. "Does Breastfeeding Empower Women? Insights from a Select Group of Educated, Low-Income, Minority Women." *Birth* 20 (1): 30–35.

Lording, Ros. 2012. "Infant Feeding: The Effects of Scheduled vs. On-Demand Feeding on Mothers' Wellbeing and Children's Cognitive Development." *Breastfeeding Review* 20 (3): 52.

Lucas, A., and T. J. Cole. 1990. "Breast Milk and Neonatal Necrotising Enterocolitis." *Lancet* 336 (8730–8731): 1519–1523.

MacDonald, Trevor, Joy Noel-Weiss, Diana West, Michelle Walks, MaryLynne Biener, Alanna Kibbe, and Elizabeth Myler. 2016. "Transmasculine Individuals' Experiences with Lactation, Chestfeeding, and Gender Identity: A Qualitative Study." *BMC Pregnancy and Childbirth* 16 (106). https://bmcpregnancychildbirth.biomedcentral.com/articles/10.1186/s12884-016-0907-y.

MacDorman, M. F., E. Declercq, and M. E. Thoma. 2017. "Trends in Maternal Mortality by Sociodemographic Characteristics and Cause of Death in 27 States and the District of Columbia." *Obstetrics and Gynecology* 129 (5): 811–818.

Mamo, Laura. 2007. *Queering Reproduction: Achieving Pregnancy in the Age of Technoscience*. Durham: Duke University Press.

Mamo, Laura, and Jennifer Ruth Fosket. 2009. "Scripting the Body: Pharmaceuticals and the (Re)Making of Menstruation." *Signs* 34 (4): 925–949.

Marshall, Joyce L., Mary Godfrey, and Mary J. Renfrew. 2007. "Being a 'Good Mother': Managing Breastfeeding and Merging Identities." *Social Science and Medicine* 65 (10): 2147–2159.

Mauthner, Natasha S. 2016. "Un/Re-making Method." In *Mattering: Feminism, Science, and Materialism*, edited by Victoria Pitts-Taylor, 258–283. New York: New York University Press.

Mayo Clinic. 2018. "Mastitis." Accessed May 23, 2018. http://www.mayoclinic.org/diseases-conditions/mastitis/basics/treatment/con-20026633.

McCarter-Spaulding, Deborah E., and Margaret H. Kearney, 2001. "Parenting Self-Efficacy and Perception of Insufficient Breast Milk." *Journal of Obstetric, Gynecologic, and Neonatal Nursing* 30 (5): 515–522.

McKenna, James J., and Lee T. Gettler. 2015. "There Is No Such Thing as Infant Sleep, There Is No Such Thing as Breastfeeding, There Is Only Breastsleeping." *Acta Paediactrica* 105 (1): 17–21.

Mead, Margaret. 1935. *Sex and Temperament in Three Primitive Societies*. New York: HarperCollins.

Medolac. n.d. "Medolac: A Public Benefit Corporation." Accessed May 23, 2018. http://www.medolac.com/page/homepage.

Mehra, B., C. Merkel, and A. P. Bishop. 2004. "The Internet for Empowerment of Minority and Marginalized Users." *New Media and Society* 6 (6): 781–802.

Mennella, J. A., C. P. Jagnow, and G. K. Beauchamp. 2001. "Prenatal and Postnatal Flavor Learning by Human Infants." *Pediatrics* 107 (6): 88.

Merewood, Anne, Supriya D. Mehta, Laura Beth Chamberlain, Barbara L. Philipp, Howard Bauchner. 2005. "Breastfeeding Rates in US Baby-Friendly Hospitals: Results of a National Survey." *Pediatrics* 116 (3): 628–634.

Milky Way Foundation, The. n.d. "Our Initiatives." Accessed May 23, 2018. http://milkywayfoundation.org/.

Mills, C. Wright. 1959. *The Sociological Imagination*. New York: Oxford University Press.

Murray, Christopher J. L., Haidong Wang, and Nicholas Kassebaum. 2016. "Sharp Decline in Maternal and Child Deaths Globally, Studies Show." *Institute for Health Metrics and Evaluation*. Accessed January 30, 2018. http://www.healthdata.org/news-release/sharp-decline-maternal-and-child-deaths-globally-new-data-show.

Murtagh, Lindsey, and Anthony D. Moulton. 2011. "Working Mothers, Breastfeeding, and the Law." *American Journal of Public Health* 101 (2): 217–223.

Naples, Nancy. 2004. "Queer Parenting in the New Millennium." *Gender and Society* 18 (6): 679–684.

Nathoo, Tasnim, and Aleck Ostry. 2010. "Wet-Nursing, Milk Banks, and Black Markets: The Political Economy of Giving Breastmilk in Canada in the 20th and 21st Century." In *Giving Breastmilk: Body Ethics and Contemporary Breastfeeding Practice*, edited by Rhonda Shaw and Alison Bartlett, 134–150. Bradford, Ontario: Demeter Press.

Nussbaum, Martha. 2011. *Creating Capabilities: The Human Development Approach*. Cambridge, Mass.: Harvard University Press.

Oparah, Julia Chinyere, and Alicia D. Bonaparte, eds. 2015. *Birthing Justice: Black Women, Pregnancy, and Childbirth*. New York: Routledge.

Palmquist, Aunchalee, and Kirsten Doehler. 2014. "Contextualizing Online Human Milk Sharing: Structural Factors and Lactation Disparity among Middle Income Women in the U.S." *Social Science and Medicine* 122:140–147.

———. 2016. "Human Milk Sharing Practices in the US." *Maternal and Child Nutrition* 12 (2): 278–290.

Park, Shelley M. 2006. "Adoptive Maternal Bodies: A Queer Paradigm for Rethinking Mothering?" *Hypatia* 21 (1): 201–226.

Pineau, Marisa Gerstein. 2011. *Liquid Gold: Breast Milk Banking in the United States*. PhD diss., University of California, Los Angeles. http://gradworks.umi.com/35/10/3510268.html.

———. 2012. "From Commodity to Donation: Breastmilk Banking in the United States from 1910 to the Present." UCLA Center for the Study of Women. http://escholarship.org/uc/item/5cq095sn#page-2.

Plummer, Ken. 2003. *Intimate Citizenship: Private Decisions and Public Dialogues*. Seattle: University of Washington Press.

Quandt, Sarah A. 1995. "Sociocultural Aspects of the Lactation Process." In *Biocultural Perspectives on Breastfeeding*, edited by Patricia Stuart-Macadam and Katherine A. Dettwyler, 127–144. New York: Aldine de Gruyter.

Raju, T. N. 2011. "Breastfeeding Is a Dynamic Biological Process—Not Simply a Meal at the Breast." *Breastfeeding Medicine* 6 (5): 257–259.

Rapp, Rayna. 2000. *Testing Women, Testing the Fetus: The Social Impact of Amniocentesis in America*. New York: Routledge.

Reich, Jennifer A. 2010. "From Maternal Love to Toxic Exposure." In *Giving Breastmilk: Body Ethics and Contemporary Breastfeeding Practice*, edited by Rhonda Shaw and Alison Bartlett, 163–174. Bradford, Ontario: Demeter Press.

———. 2011. "Public Mothers and Private Practices: Breastfeeding as Transgression." In *Embodied Resistance: Challenging the Norms, Breaking the Rules*, edited by Chris Bobel and Samantha Kwan, 130–142. Nashville: Vanderbilt University Press.

———. 2016. *Calling the Shots: Why Parents Reject Vaccines*. New York: New York University Press.

Rey, K. R., E. P. Davis, C. A. Sandman, and L. M. Glynn. 2013. "Human Milk Cortisol Is Associated with Infant Temperament." *Psychoneuroendocrinology* 38 (7): 1178–1185.

Reyes-Foster, Beatriz, Shannon K. Carter, and Hinajosa Melanie Sbrena. 2015. "Milk Sharing in Practice: A Descriptive Analysis of Breast Milk Sharing." *Breastfeeding Medicine* 10 (5): 263–269.

Rich, Adrienne. 1976. *Of Woman Born: Motherhood as Experience and as Institution*. New York: W. W. Norton.

Roberts, Dorothy. 1997. *Killing the Black Body: Race, Reproduction, and the Meaning of Liberty*. New York: Vintage Books.

Rothman, Barbara Katz. 1989. "Women as Fathers: Motherhood and Child Care under a Modified Patriarchy." *Gender and Society* 3 (1): 89–104.

———. (1989) 2000. *Recreating Motherhood*. Brunswick: Rutgers University Press.

———. 2007. "Laboring Now: Current Cultural Constructions of Pregnancy, Birth, and Mothering." In *Laboring On: Birth in Transition in the United States*, edited by Wendy Simonds, Barbara Katz Rothman, and Bari Meltzer Norman, 29–96. New York: Routledge.

———. 2016. *A Bun in the Oven: How the Food and Birth Movements Resist Medicalization*. New York: New York University Press.

Rudrappa, Sharmila. 2015. *Discounted Life: The Price of Global Surrogacy in India*. New York: New York University Press.

Ryan, Kath, Paul Bissell, and Jo Alexander. 2010. "Moral Work in Women's Narratives of Breastfeeding." *Social Science and Medicine* 70 (6): 951–958.

Ryan, Kath, Victoria Team, and Jo Alexander. 2013. "Expressionists of the 21st Century: The Commodification and Commercialization of the Expressed Breast Milk." *Medical Anthropology* 32 (5): 467–486.

Ryan, Kath, Les Todres, and Jo Alexander. 2010. "Calling, Permission, and Fulfillment: The Interembodied Experience of Breastfeeding." *Qualitative Health Research* 21 (6): 731–742.

Saha, Moni R., Kath Ryan, and Lisa H. Amir. 2015. "Postpartum Women's Use of Medicines and Breastfeeding Practices: A Systematic Review." *International Breastfeeding* 10 (1): 28.

Said, Edward. 1978. *Orientalism*. New York: Vintage Books.

Salamon, Gayle, 2010. *Assuming a Body: Transgender and Rhetorics of Materiality*. New York: Columbia University Press.

Schmied, Virginia, and Deborah Lupton. 2001. "Blurring the Boundaries: Breastfeeding and Subjectivity." *Sociology of Health and Illness* 23 (2): 234–250.

Scrinis, Gyorgy. 2013. *Nutritionism: The Science and Politics of Dietary Advice*. New York: Columbia University Press.

Seidman, Steven. 1995. "Deconstructing Queer Theory or the Under-Theorization of the Social and the Ethical." In *Social Postmodernism: Beyond Identity Politics*, edited by Linda Nicholson and Steven Seidman, 116–141. Cambridge, U.K.: Cambridge University Press.

Shaw, Rhonda M. 2007. "Cross-Nursing, Ethics, and Giving Breastmilk in the Contemporary Context." *Women's Studies International Forum* 30 (5): 439–450.

———. 2010. "Perspectives on Ethics and Human Milk Banking." In *Giving Breastmilk: Body Ethics and Contemporary Breastfeeding Practices*, edited by Rhonda M. Shaw and Alison Bartlett, 83–97. Bradford, Ontario: Demeter Press.

Shaw, Rhonda M., and Robert Webb. 2015. "Multiple Meanings of 'Gift' and Its Value for Organ Donation." *Qualitative Health Research* 25 (5): 600–611.

Sheff, Elisabeth. 2013. *The Polyamorists Next Door: Inside Multiple-Partner Relationships and Families*. Lanham: Rowman and Littlefield.

Shim, Jeun, JuHee Kim, and Rose Ann Mathai. 2011. "Associations of Infant Feeding Practices and Picky Eating Behaviors of Preschool Children." *Journal of the Academy of Nutrition and Dietetics* 111 (9): 1363–1368.

Simonds, Wendy. 2002. "Watching the Clock: Keeping Time during Pregnancy, Birth, and Postpartum Experiences." *Social Science and Medicine* 55 (4): 559–570.

Simonds, Wendy, Barbara Katz Rothman, and Bari Meltzer Norman. 2007. *Laboring On: Birth in Transition in the United States*. New York: Routledge.

Smyth, Lisa. 2008. "Gendered Spaces and Intimate Citizenship: The Case of Breastfeeding." *European Journal of Women's Studies* 15 (2): 83–99.

Stacey, Judith. 1988. "Can There Be a Feminist Ethnography?" *Women's Studies International Forum* 11 (1): 21–27.

Stanford, Acquanda Y. 2016. "Uncovering Imperialist White Supremacist Capitalist Patriarchy in Professional Breastfeeding Services: The Greater Complexities of IBCLCs." *Acquanda Y. Stanford* (blog), May 19, 2016. Accessed May 23, 2018. http://acquandastanford.com/uncovering-imperialist-white-supremacist-capitalist -patriarchy-in-professional-breastfeeding-services-the-greater-complexities-of -ibclcs/.

Stearns, Cindy. 2010. "The Breast Pump." In *Giving Breastmilk: Body Ethics and Contemporary Breastfeeding Practice*, edited by Rhonda Shaw and Alison Bartlett, 11–23. Bradford, Ontario: Demeter Press.

Stuart-Macadam, Patricia, and Katherine A. Dettwyler, eds. 1995. *Biocultural Perspectives on Breastfeeding*. New York: Aldine de Gruyter.

Stuebe, Alison. 2014. "Enabling Women to Achieve Their Breastfeeding Goals." *Obstetrics and Gynecology* 123 (3): 643–652.

Svanborg, C., H. Ågerstam, A. Aronson, R. Bjerkvig, C. Düringer, W. Fischer, L. Gustafsson, O. Hallgren, I. Leijonhuvud, S. Linse, and A. K. Mossberg. 2003. "HAMLET Kills Tumor Cells by an Apoptosis-Like Mechanism—Cellular, Molecular, and Therapeutic Aspects." *Advances in Cancer Research* 88:1–29.

Tomori, Cecilia. 2014. *Nighttime Breastfeeding: An American Cultural Dilemma*. New York: Berghahn Books.

Tomori, Cecilia, Aunchalee E. L. Palmquist, and Sally Dowling. 2016. "Negotiating Breastfeeding Stigma in Breastmilk Sharing, Nighttime Breastfeeding, and Long-Term Breastfeeding in the U.S. and the U.K." *Social Science and Medicine* 168:178–185.

Torres, Jennifer M.C. 2014. "Medicalizing to Demedicalize: Lactation Consultants and the (De)Medicalization of Breastfeeding." *Social Science and Medicine* 100:159–166.

Tsing, Anna L. 2005. *Friction: An Ethnography of Global Connection*. Princeton: Princeton University Press.

Tuteur, Amy. 2016a. *Push Back: Guilt in the Age of Natural Parenting*. New York: Dey Street Books.

———. 2016b. "The Baby Friendly Hospital Initiative Is Like Abstinence-Only Sex Education." *The Skeptical OB* (blog), July 14, 2016. Accessed May 23, 2018. http://www.skepticalob.com/2016/07/the-baby-friendly-hospital-initiative-is-like-abstinence-only-sex-education.html.

U.S. Department of Health and Human Services. 2011. "The Surgeon General's Call to Action to Support Breastfeeding." Washington, D.C.: U.S. Department of Health and Human Services, Office of the Surgeon General. http://www.surgeongeneral.gov.

U.S. National Library of Medicine. 2018. "Lactose Intolerance." Genetics Home Reference (website). Accessed May 23, 2018. https://ghr.nlm.nih.gov/condition/lactose-intolerance#statistics.

Van Esterik, Penny. 2010. "Breastfeeding and HIV/AIDS: Critical Gaps and Dangerous Intersections." In *Giving Breastmilk: Body Ethics and Contemporary Breastfeeding Practice*, edited by Rhonda Shaw and Alison Bartlett, 151–162. Bradford, Ontario: Demeter Press.

Viveiros de Castro, Eduardo. 2013. "The Relative Native." Translated by Julia Saama and Martin Holbraad. *Journal of Ethnographic Theory* 3 (3): 469.

Vohr, B. R., B. B. Poindexter, A. M. Dusick, L. T. McKinley, L. L. Wright, J. C. Langer, and W. K. Poole. 2006. "Beneficial Effects of Breast Milk in the Neonatal Intensive Care Unit on the Developmental Outcome of Extremely Low Birth Weight Infants at 18 Months of Age." *Pediatrics* 118 (1): 115–123. http://dx.doi.org/10.1438/hau3.3.033.

Waldman, Ayelet. 2009. *Bad Mother: A Chronicle of Maternal Crimes, Minor Calamities, and Occasional Moments of Grace*. New York: Anchor Books.

Wall, Glenda. 2001. "Moral Constructions of Motherhood in Breastfeeding Discourse." *Gender and Society* 15 (4): 592–610.

Waltz, Miriam. 2014. "Milk and Management: Breastfeeding as a Project." *Anthropology Journal, Southern Africa* 37 (1–2): 42–49.

Weasel, Lisa H. 2016. "Embodying Intersectionality." In *Mattering: Feminism, Science, and Materialism*, edited by Victoria Pitts-Taylor, 104–121. Durham: Duke University Press.

Welter, Barbara. 1966. "The Cult of True Womanhood, 1820–1860." *American Quarterly* 2 (1): 151–174.

West, Candace, and Don H. Zimmerman. 1987. "Doing Gender." *Gender and Society* 1 (2): 125–151.

Weston A. Price Foundation. 2018. "About the Weston A. Price Foundation." Accessed May 23, 2018. http://www.westonaprice.org/.

Whalen, Bonny, and Rachel Cramton. 2010. "Overcoming Barriers to Breastfeeding Continuation and Exclusivity." *Pediatrics* 22 (5): 655–663.

Wiley, Andrea S. 2016. *Re-imagining Milk: Cultural and Biological Perspectives.* 2nd ed. New York: Routledge.

Wolf, Jacqueline H. 2001. *Don't Kill Your Baby: Public Health and the Decline of Breastfeeding in the 19th and 20th Centuries.* Columbus: Ohio State University Press.

Wolf, Joan B. 2011. *Is Breast Best? Taking on the Breastfeeding Experts and the New High Stakes of Motherhood.* New York: New York University Press.

Zeigler, John B., Richard O. Johnson, David A. Cooper, and Julian Gold. 1985. "Postnatal Transmission of Aids-Associated Retrovirus from Mother to Infant." *Lancet* 8434: 896–898.

Zizzo, Gabriella. 2009. "Lesbian Families and the Negotiation of Maternal Identity through the Unconventional Use of Breast Milk." *Gay and Lesbian Issues and Psychology Review* 5 (2): 96–109.

INDEX

ABOUT THE AUTHOR

KRISTIN J. WILSON is chair of the Anthropology Department at Cabrillo College. She is the author of *Not Trying: Infertility, Childlessness, and Ambivalence* (2014) published by Vanderbilt University Press. She previously taught in the Sociology Department of Georgia State University and worked as an ethnographer at the Rollins School of Public Health at Emory University in Atlanta.